T3-AIB-840

155.412 Kes
Kestenberg.
The role of movement
 patterns in development.

The Lorette Wilmot Library
Nazareth College of Rochester

The Role of Movement Patterns in Development

Vol. 1

by
Judith S. Kestenberg, M.D.

DISCARDED
LORETTE WILMOT LIBRARY
NAZARETH COLLEGE

NEW YORK 1977  DANCE NOTATION BUREAU PRESS

© 1967, by Psychoanalytic Quarterly, Inc.
Second Printing, April 1971

This is an unabridged republication by the
Dance Notation Bureau
19 Union Square West
New York, N.Y. 10003

TABLE OF CONTENTS

LIST OF ILLUSTRATIONS

THE ROLE OF MOVEMENT PATTERNS IN DEVELOPMENT

I. RHYTHMS OF MOVEMENT

BY JUDITH S. KESTENBERG, M.D. (NEW YORK)

Pleasure and unpleasure, therefore, cannot be referred to an increase or decrease of a quantity (which we describe as 'tension due to stimulus'), although they obviously have a great deal to do with that factor. It appears that they depend, not on this quantitative factor, but on some characteristic of it which we can only describe as a qualitative one. If we were able to say what this qualitative characteristic is, we should be much further advanced in psychology. Perhaps it is the rhythm, the temporal sequence of changes, rises and falls in the quantity of the stimulus. We do not know (21, p. 160).

THE CONTRIBUTIONS OF FREUD AND FERENCZI

The problem of excitation, tension, and discharge occurs often in Freud's writings (for instance, [18, 19, 20, 22]). Many of his theorizations about instinctual drives and instinctual energy are based not only on neurophysiological models but on direct observations of movement as well. Breuer and Freud's concept of 'tonic intracerebral excitation', operative in the waking state, seems to be derived from the clinically observable tonus of muscles at rest (18). The closely allied concept of bound and free energy, which pervades Freud's later theories, may well have been influenced by observations of tonic and clonic movements familiar to neurologists. Observations of muscular tensions and relaxations during certain affective and ideational states may have been a further source of Freud's theory of energy.

From the Department of Psychiatry, Division of Psychoanalytic Education, State University of New York, Downstate Medical Center, Brooklyn, New York.

Ferenczi contrasted the expression of emotions in which explosion predominates with those in which inhibition prevails *(13)*. Some years later he described thinkers who inhibited their motility in order to think. These, he believed, contrasted with 'rapid thinkers who move around in order to retard the overwhelming onrush of their ideas' *(14)*. Ferenczi appeared to be in agreement with Freud when he wrote: 'The regular parallelism of motor innervations with the psychic acts of thinking and attention, their mutual conditioning, and frequently demonstrable quantitative reciprocity, speak at any rate for an essential similarity in these processes' *(14,* p. 231*)*.

Freud and Breuer used their clinical observations of individual predilections for certain motor patterns as an index of differences in the nervous systems of individuals. They wrote: 'We are familiar with the great individual variations which are found in this respect: the great differences between lively people and inert and lethargic ones, between those who "cannot sit still" and those who have an "innate gift for lounging on sofas", and between mentally agile minds and dull ones which can tolerate intellectual rests for an unlimited length of time. These differences which make up a man's natural temperament are certainly based on profound differences in his nervous system—on the degree to which the functionally quiescent cerebral elements liberate energy' *(18)*.

RECENT STUDIES OF MOTILITY

As analysts' interest shifted from the drives to the ego functions, they have laid aside the early theories based on neurophysiology and on observation of movements. Study of character formation has occupied psychoanalytic thought ever since, whereas research on temperament, as expressed in both motor patterns and styles of thinking, has become almost obsolete. Yet the concept of discharge of psychic energy has remained important.

Papers concerned with rhythmic and nonrhythmic pattern of motor discharge have been few. Kris *(33)*, in a study of laughter, said that 'in states of sensuous excitement everything presses forward with a different rhythm'. He quoted Glover's statement that the motor apparatus functions in many ways reminiscent of infantile motility *(26)*. Since the id 'has no expressive behavior', Kris postulated that only ego controls can alter primitive forms of rhythmicity into mimetic expressiveness. When the ego is overwhelmed by instinctual forces, a breakthrough of rhythmicity becomes evident in the shaking of laughter, in uncontrollable crying and sobbing. This type of rhythm, Kris pointed out, differs from rhythmic motility controlled by the ego. Perhaps we may restate the opinion of Kris as follows: the primitive rhythm of affective discharge as it is modified by the ego becomes a vehicle for nonverbal communication.

Kris' attempt to delineate the regulatory influence of the ego upon the primitive rhythmic discharge in laughter remained a unique contribution to the study of hierarchy of functions and change of functions (Hartmann [*28*]) until Erikson classified successive modes of ego organization, derived from drive discharge patterns *(10, 11)*. In 1952, Jacobson *(29)* examined the pace of psychic discharge processes and subsequently Greenacre *(27)* distinguished two types of rhythm in infantile motility. Piaget examined one aspect of the rhythmic quality of neonatal movements *(40)*. He pointed out that the early rhythms, such as the alternating opening and closing of the mouth, observable in the neonate, are given up in favor of a 'regulation' which controls later more complex behavior. Unfortunately Piaget did not pursue the study of motor rhythms and regulations of motility.

Although both academic and psychoanalytic developmental psychology are based in good part on observation of motor behavior, no systematic study of rhythms of motor discharge has been attempted. Deutsch *(6, 7, 8, 9)* analyzed posture and movement chiefly as they relate to the understanding of the subject's hidden thoughts. Fries *(23, 24, 25)* was the first analyst who tried to relate early motor behavior with later psychic manifestations. Her classification of temperaments as 'active', 'moderately active', and 'quiet', however, did not take into account the individuality of the motor rhythm. She did convey the impression that characteristic, though not well-defined, motor patterns are detectable in early infancy. Many subsequent studies have shown that one of the most important differences between early and later behavior is in motility *(1, 5, 12, 16, 17, 38, 39, 40, 42, 43, 44)*. But the lack of classification of infantile and adult qualities of movement made it difficult to compare early and later forms of motor behavior. Motor development has been primarily appraised by tests of specific achievements such as grasping or sitting, rather than of qualities or sequences of movement.

CLASSIFICATION OF MOVEMENT

About ten years ago I initiated a pilot study for the classification of movement. Three infants were observed and tested in the nursery and later at home.[1] General behavioral data were recorded with the aim of correlating them with corresponding movement patterns. Early recordings of movements were descriptive. Later recordings consisted of freehand tracings of the rise and fall of the flow of movements. Eventually the movement assessment method, as originated by Laban and developed by Lamb, was used *(2, 3, 34, 35, 36)*. While Laban's test was geared to the study of adaptive motility, the tracing of the rise and fall of flow was useful for the study of motor rhythms.

Rhythm notation consists of the recorder's freehand drawing of the increase and decrease of muscle tension during movement. It is based on the observer's kinesthetic mirroring identification with the observed subject. The tracing must be done

[1] Dr. Jacqueline Friend observed and tested the children regularly from the ages of three to twelve months; Dr. Stephanie Librach took over this task for several months of their second year. Dr. Sibylle Escalona tested them at fourteen months and Dr. Florence Halpern did so just before and during late latency. Irma Bartenieff recorded their movements several times in the years of latency. I am indebted to these investigators for their observations and evaluations.

with free-floating attention while at the same time one has to judge the rate of increase of tension, the degree of the intensity reached, and the frequency of fluctuations of tension during a given sequence of movement. One must note whether the tension of agonistic and antagonistic muscles is such that the movement appears inhibited or the relaxation of the antagonists has led to free motor discharge (32). The attitude of free-floating attention is tempered by these considerations as well as by the recorder's awareness of her own preferences for certain rhythms which tend to distort kinesthetic perception and reproduction of another person's movements. (Note the similarity to countertransference.)

In the beginning of the study, it was possible to observe motor rhythms in gratification, frustration, random movements, and play. After the first year the data on gratification and frustration rhythms were not readily available. But the increasing availability of verbally communicated psychic content made it possible to study the correlation between ideation and rhythms of motor discharge.

The following two reports focus on the description and interpretation of motor rhythms. The preliminary report, which covers the time of the neonatal period to nine months, was originally written in collaboration with Dr. Jacqueline Friend and was presented at the Arden House Conference in 1954 (see Anna Freud's discussion [15]). In. this preliminary report an attempt was made to correlate the behavior of infants and their mothers with changes in the infants' patterns of movement. Intuitive predictions formulated at that time will be re-examined later in this paper where the follow-up study, covering data accumulated during almost ten years of periodic observation and testing, is discussed.

PRELIMINARY REPORT OF THREE INFANTS

Rhythms of infantile movement seem to be determined by a congenital pattern. Preferences for certain rhythms may persist into adulthood even though movement becomes more complex as the nervous system matures. As the child grows up, fantasies provide content, add purpose so to speak to forms of excitation and discharge congenitally determined.

The infant is likely to respond to stimuli from the outside world as he does to stimuli from within. Sequences of excitation, gratification, and relaxation, which are dictated by inner needs, may be inappropriate for successful adaptation to the environment. If such 'undesirable' patterns are encouraged they may become fixed, indelible foundations of personality traits. But premature consistent interference with congenitally preferred motor patterns may retard development or enhance the early formation of rigid defenses. In either case we observe the beginnings of later pathology in the first year of life. Fortunately the early disturbances are often overcome, not only because young children respond quickly to better handling, but also because even if the environment does not improve, the infant is often able to recover by use of his own resources. Especially in the latter part of the first year the child becomes increasingly able to learn from his own experiences, achieving relative independence from the adults in charge of him. He is often successful in finding his own solutions, which may represent only slight modifications of the original pattern yet do not bring him into conflict with the demands of the environment. Children unable to recover may join the ranks of the many so-called borderline adults whose dealing with reality is forever precarious. Sometimes after analyzing and working through innumerable layers of the fantasies of such adults, we are still confronted with the same repetitive 'undesirable pattern'—a form without content.

'Form without content' is more simply explained by the Polish psychologist, Janusz Korczak. Whether they are Franks or Shmuls, he wrote, children fall into three distinct categories when presented with a dish of potatoes and scrambled eggs. The first type eats the scrambled eggs first and is left with the dreary potatoes for the end; the second type eats the potatoes first, keeping the scrambled eggs to the last possible moment; and the third wisely mixes the potatoes and scrambled eggs, thus enjoying both throughout the meal.

The three children we observed seem to fit Korczak's classification of types. Each of the children had a decided preference for certain forms of motor discharge which could be noted not only in such excitation-gratification-relaxation cycles as occur before, during, and after nursing but also in random activity, play, and early achievement. Greenacre (27) has contrasted rhythms of gratification with those of 'lolling' movements in infants. A similar but not identical subdivision will be used in this report; namely, 'gratification' rhythms and 'functional pleasure' rhythms (30, 31). In our three subjects these rhythms were intrinsically related to each other. The motor patterns during activities giving functional pleasure appeared to be miniature duplications of the more intense rhythmic discharge during periods of excitation, gratification, and relaxation (see Illustration 1).

Illustration 1. A. "Gratification" rhythm.
B. "Functional Pleasure" Rhythm.

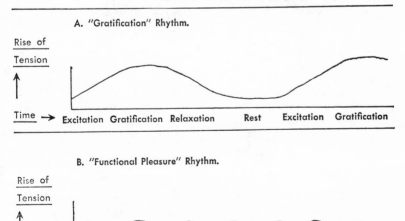

A. "Gratification" Rhythm.

Rise of Tension

Time → Excitation Gratification Relaxation Rest Excitation Gratification

B. "Functional Pleasure" Rhythm.

Rise of Tension

Time → Rest Rest Rest Rest Rest Rest Rest

I

Glenda resembled Korczak's first type, who ate the scrambled eggs first and then the potatoes. From the start she drank her milk for a short time only; her initial interest quickly waning, she would fall asleep and cease to suck. Her mother was able to feed her frequently, but briefly. When the time came to spoon-feed her, she was presented with spoonfuls in rapid succession so that feeding time was still a brief affair. Glenda showed extreme agility from birth. In the hospital she would propel herself to the very end of her bassinet. She did this lying on her back, a feat that provoked admiration not only from the nurses but also from people visiting other babies. She propelled herself by successive cycles of leg motions and rest periods. When, after several alternations of motion and rest, she arrived at the head of the bassinet and could move no farther, she would cry.

Soon after Glenda went home, her mother recognized the infant's need to move in the crib and ceased covering her tightly. As a result of this understanding between mother and child, Glenda was able to develop freely and became extraordinarily resourceful when left to her own devices. When she was nine months old, she fell while trying to climb a rocking chair; the chair fell on her and imprisoned her underneath. She gave the observer a look as if to say 'help me', but when no help was given, with some effort she turned face down, lifting the chair as she did so. After a satisfied moment of rest, and giving the observer another brief look, she attempted to sit down which partially freed her foot. Again she rested, playing with the chair and examining a toy which had fallen from it. Then she turned her attention to her still imprisoned foot, and with a sudden movement freed this foot too.

Although at first it had seemed that Glenda was a child who gave up quickly, it was clear later that she did not give up for good, but merely needed frequent periods of relaxation between spurts of activity. Her mother started prohibitions early and these soon became quite effective during certain phases of her cycles of excitation and relaxation. She adopted the moments of prohibited activity as her rest periods, experiencing them, it seemed, as pleasant interruptions (or, better, as interpolations) quite in keeping with one phase of her preferred rhythm. When the prohibitions were not given at the start of an activity, they did not seem to represent interferences or interruptions. At nine months, for example, Glenda was creeping to the bathroom. When she came close to it, her mother told her not to go there. She immediately stopped creeping, sat down, and looked at her mother pleasantly. After a short interval, she proceeded to creep in the forbidden direction again. But an admonition that coincided with the onset of her creeping had no effect.

Two changes in rhythm which later became noticeable did not seem to be related to maternal interventions. Glenda's periods of rest became even shorter than before, perhaps because of an increase in motor impulses. On the other hand, Glenda became cautious at times. Instead of suddenly plopping down from standing, she now released her hold on the supporting object, such as a chair, more gradually. Through her own experience of climbing and falling she may have learned that sudden drops in muscle tension are followed by displeasure. Glenda's preferred motor rhythms can be represented graphically.

Illustration 2. Glenda's preferred rhythm

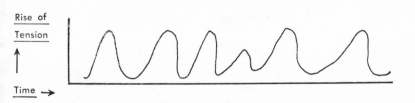

Rise of

Tension

↑

Time →

To be more precise the observed rhythms would be sub-divided as follows:

Illustration 3. Subdivision of Glenda's
rhythms at nine months.

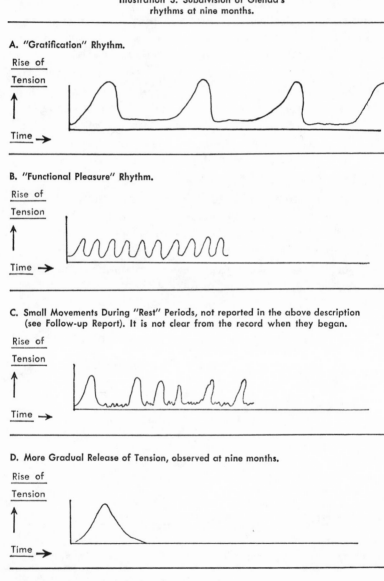

A. "Gratification" Rhythm.

Rise of
Tension

Time →

B. "Functional Pleasure" Rhythm.

Rise of
Tension

Time →

C. Small Movements During "Rest" Periods, not reported in the above description (see Follow-up Report). It is not clear from the record when they began.

Rise of
Tension

Time →

D. More Gradual Release of Tension, observed at nine months.

Rise of
Tension

Time →

Glenda was a well baby, relatively free of conflict even though she preferred a pattern of motor discharge that began abruptly and ceased prematurely, not permitting prolonged uninterrupted activity. Despite a serious sickness at the age of five months, which led to hospitalization for several days and separation from her mother, Glenda steadily progressed in her development and was a happy, contented, normal child.

The other two infants showed behavior destined to become pathological.

II

Nancy roughly resembled Korczak's second type: she might keep her scrambled eggs until the last minute. She was quite hungry in the hospital and her formula had to be increased several times in her first few days of life. Long before feeding time she would cry, move about, and only briefly find some satisfaction. When nursing from the bottle she did not appear avid, but showed signs of great enjoyment. Soon after feeding, however, she seemed dissatisfied. She acted as if satiation was never possible.

Her movements gave the impression of an irregular staccato rhythm. Even in what seemed to be peace, there was an irregular increase of tonus.[2] Her period of excitement was long and her relaxation short. She cried soon after her feeding. When put on her belly, she made irregular locomotor strides and would end up at the head of the bassinet, rooting with her mouth like a puppy in search of food. For this type of locomotion her good tonus served her well. In contrast to Glenda who moved like a dancer, Nancy jerked, pushed, and went on and on relentlessly.

---

[2]Tonus is used for lack of a better term; it pertains by definition to the state of muscle tension at rest. A better term might be 'bound flow' which adequately describes Nancy's main characteristic. The concepts of bound and free flow will be introduced in a subsequent paper *(32)*.

She seemed to be in a perpetual cramp except when deeply asleep for a brief period shortly after feeding. In a frantic way she would maneuver her head and arms until she sometimes got her hand into her mouth; occasionally she would hold one hand with the other in order to accomplish this. Complete relaxation would then ensue just as after feeding, but soon her hand would fall out and the struggle would begin again; she would stiffen, cry, and appear to 'seek' with head, mouth, and hands.

Nancy's curve of excitation, gratification, and relaxation might be drawn as follows:

Illustration 4. Nancy's "rhythmicity".

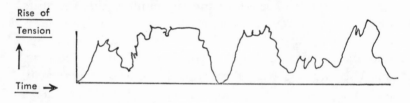

Rise of
Tension

↑

Time →

Nancy's mother responded to her urgent need by appeasing her quickly, not allowing her to cry. But no sooner did the child get home from the nursery than feedings by her mother ceased. Her bottle was propped on a pillow and the baby was left to fend for herself. When she lost the nipple, she sometimes retrieved it but at other times could not. Whether by natural inclination or because of the frustration caused by losing the nipple, Nancy would fall asleep holding the nipple in her mouth. When grasping developed the mother handed her two spoons; Nancy would hold a spoon in each hand for most of the day and sometimes even during the night.

The prop-feeding prevented Nancy's moving around much. Lying on her back all the time, she soon started to raise her head and maintain this position for long periods. She was slow to sit without support because she attempted to sit stiffly, raising her head and trunk; this exposed her to the danger of losing her balance and falling backward like a board. She was unable to creep in a normal fashion, probably because she had hardly any practice in the prone position. When at eight months she finally jerked herself around onto her buttocks and propelled herself grotesquely on one thigh, her mother was amused.

Nancy's mother discouraged her moving about but urged her to rock rather violently, in a way reminiscent of the forceful pushing forward in her earliest months.[3] Although she cried easily and could be consoled only by being picked up by a member of the family, her mother considered her a peaceful, untroubled child. Nancy's facial expression, however, seemed tense, anxious, and sad. Her motor retardation, peculiar locomotion, and inability to play with objects did not worry the family.

The mother's frequent prohibitions and commands, such as 'stop crying', 'rock, Nancy, rock', or 'stop rocking', were absorbed in the numerous tension states of the child's sequence of excitation and relaxation. These prohibitions and commands became rigidly enforced and fixed. The degree of Nancy's obedience was demonstrated, for example, when her mother forbade her to interfere with the eating utensils during feeding. Soon thereafter Nancy, aged eight months, was being fed her favorite custard, in each hand holding a spoon while her mother fed her with a third spoon. When, at the observer's suggestion, her mother removed the two spoons from Nancy's hands and the observer offered her the feeding spoon, she would not reach for it. Her arm and face stiffened. She withdrew her arm from the spoon when it was brought nearer to her hand, apparently not only unable to accept it but also actively avoiding it.

At nine months there was a change in Nancy's behavior. She still looked stiff and tense but she now was able to release ob-

[3] In retrospect we must note that neither rocking nor pushing were done with force but rather by an alternation of explosiveness and inhibition which gave the observer an impression of forceful violence.

jects. After her return home from the hospital soon after birth, her stiffness and tension had increased considerably so that her newfound ability to relax and release was the more striking. She seemed so fascinated by this experience of release that she even used it while eating. She would drop her lower jaw and let food spill out of her mouth, despite her obvious enjoyment of it. There was however a peculiar quality to her movements of release. They were almost casual, slow, and meek, giving the impression of involuntary movements in absentmindedness.[4]

Nancy's environment steadily supported her tendency to hold on tensely. Unless her ability to relax, which she developed at nine months, could free her from the pervasive tonic pattern, her subsequent development could be expected to be further hampered by lack of practice and her personality to suffer from an unusual rigidity of ego and superego.

III

From the start Charlie impressed one as likely to be the type who mixes potatoes with scrambled eggs (Korczak's third example). Particularly noticeable were the intensity and persistence with which he responded and his unusual ability to absorb and enjoy experiences ordinarily felt as unpleasant, frustrating interruptions. The impression of persistence and intensity was created by a smooth, gradual increase of excitement that would not deviate from its course despite disturbing stimuli and would rise to a high plateau.

During nursing Charlie made sounds of delight of an orgastic quality. He would persevere in drinking unusually steadily

---

[4] Even as a neonate Nancy could pass from stiffness to limpness. Glenda at nine months had learned to inhibit her preferred explosive discharge while Nancy at the same age was going from the extreme of cramping, not to controlled release but to limpness, which only accidentally produced release. Thus Nancy did not really acquire control; she merely relinquished inhibition.

for prolonged periods, all the while watching the constant coming and going of his family and neighbors. If he stopped drinking for a moment, he did so only because he needed to 'burp'. It took some time to release the bubble; this prompted his mother to call him stubborn. Charlie ordinarily gave the impression of great composure, even in frustration, but once he reached the limit of his endurance he became inconsolable. He would cry steadily and uninterruptedly with the same intensity and endurance seen when he experienced gratification.

Whether Charlie nursed happily, cried in frustration, played, or practiced early motor skills such as grasping, his excitement would rise gradually and steadily. He seemed placid. There was nothing abrupt or explosive about him, but his excitement would rise more quickly and was subject to more fluctuations when he was stimulated by his mother. When his mother tried to get him to 'talk' to her, she would nod and vocalize in a rhythm characterized by abruptness and by frequent changes in intensity. Charlie responded with a quicker arousal than was usual for him. His motility seemed to mirror his mother's fluctuating pace. When only a few weeks old, he 'talked' back to his mother with great excitement. His face would get red, his trunk and neck would strain forward toward her as he vocalized in response to her voice and movement. His excitement would not cease when the stimulation stopped. When she did not return to his side he became frustrated much quicker than was usual for him.

The change in rhythm of motor discharge which Charlie displayed in response to his mother may have been due to his natural tendency to arouse more quickly in response to the type of rhythm with which she stimulated him. It may have been even then an adaptation of rate of arousal to better mirror his mother's excitation pattern. His usual rhythm of motor discharge and the modification of it in response to his mother's stimulation are illustrated as follows.

Illustration 5. Charlie's rhythms. A. Preferred Rhythm.
B. Modified rhythm in response to maternal stimulation.

A. Preferred Rhythm.

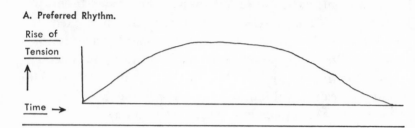

B. Modified Rhythm in response to maternal stimulation.

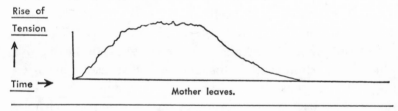

Charlie sat up early and was skilful in reaching for toys. He was used to being fed or bathed in a very busy, noisy kitchen where he also sat in a low chair and played. Occasionally he would stare ahead with 'glassy' eyes in a manner that suggested that he was then oblivious to his surroundings. By the time he reached six months, Charlie, who had been able to absorb a variety of stimuli and could enjoy many experiences simultaneously, began to show signs of shock and withdrawal. He refused to reach for toys and protested when he was taken into the kitchen. He preferred to be left alone in the crib where he played peacefully with his hands and feet, for which he reached quite well. He drank his milk less happily than before. By the time he was seven months old, he refused solids, especially while teething. Even at nine months when there was beginning evidence of recovery, his mother found it impossible to feed him solids except when he was ready to accept them. No coaxing and no distraction helped. This 'negative' period taught the family a lesson: no one can force Charlie.

Yet it would be incorrect to say that Charlie was negative and withdrawn during the few months he refused to mingle with others and preferred to be by himself in his crib. When one approached him there in a friendly way, he still smiled broadly and talked his baby language. If one did not insist that he reach for toys while sitting, he could be coaxed to do so after a while. But he would choose the toy he liked and play with it when he felt like doing so, and not when it was offered to him. The observer was able to feed him solids at the time he refused them from his mother. He would not take the spoon when it was brought to his lips but he would move his mouth toward it if it was patiently held in front of him. Feeding him at his own time and speed took a tremendous amount of time, which his busy mother could not possibly give him. Treated in ways acceptable to him, Charlie responded well; he withdrew only when approached in a different manner.

What went wrong? Why did Charlie give up activity he had started to enjoy? We can only guess. There are probably several cumulative reasons for his regression. His enjoyment of oral gratification was spoiled by the introduction of solids, which was preceded by an earlier habit of propping the bottle for him rather than holding him. The solids may have been distasteful because of the impatient, quick way his mother fed him. This very intelligent, alert mother had neither time nor patience to feed in her arms a child who took over half an hour for most feedings. The quick succession of spoonfuls presented to him was more than he could endure. He could absorb interruptions but he could not accept hurrying. He protested against solids after a while by moving his head away and spitting. He refused toys because of the chaotic way they were given to him. Several toys were pushed at him at once, and quickly taken away before he had a chance to decide which one to take. Almost all toys were too large for his grip. To top it all, Charlie began to suffer intensely from teething and no relief was offered for his aching gums. Putting his hands in his mouth was discouraged early and he did not seem to find his way back to it. Yet in other respects his mother could fulfil his needs very well. She would stimulate him vocally by an excited sing-song way of talking. The fact that he reacted to her intensely, rising to a high and persistent peak, was a source of great pleasure for her. His good relation to his mother did not really change during the period of self-imposed solitude. He gave up performing except at his own rhythm and still did not lose his broad, friendly smile when approached in the right way. He seemed to develop a successful method of passive resistance against interference with his own mode of life. Furthermore, he needed peace to cope with the pain in his gums. By nine months he already had six teeth and another one coming. It is possible that the experience of repeated relief from pain after each eruption of a tooth contributed greatly to his newfound ability at nine months to assert himself without having to resort to withdrawal and regression. He now wanted to sit with others and cried when someone took a toy away from him. He still refused solids most of the time. He evolved a 'no' gesture which he used well, although not always appropriately. He began to fight for his own rights which his active family had to respect.

Charlie's curve of excitation-gratification-relaxation did not change in the period of withdrawal. He merely refused gratification that did not conform to his pattern. His placidity and relaxation remained essentially the same. His old tenacity was used successfully in his insistence on withdrawal. After the period of withdrawal was over, his ability to absorb and enjoy several stimuli at once was not lost. He became, however, very selective in what he enjoyed, but continued his interest in various activities that required synthesis and organization. He became an excellent imitator and a good learner. He played pat-a-cake very easily, but only if his mother kept a certain rhythm in reciting the jingle to him. He refused to fall asleep unless his mother sang a special pat-a-cake tune at his bedtime.

Despite all the efforts of those about him to bend Charlie's rhythm to fit theirs, he seemed to remain basically unchanged in temperament. The tenacity and rigidity with which he held onto his innate rhythm led to early conflicts. For a while it seemed that withdrawal and restriction of his ego would result, but instead he came out of these conflicts with his environment with signs of an ego development ahead of that of Glenda, the healthy child.

As we completed our nine-month observation of Glenda, Nancy, and Charlie, we made predictions—or perhaps we should say, asked ourselves questions—about the future development of the three children.

'Were it not for a number of complicating factors, omitted here for the sake of clarity, we might be able to predict the ideational content to which these early patterns may lend themselves in the future. Will Glenda develop a strong penis envy which will be quite difficult to resolve because she will only give it up for short periods to resume her fight for it again and again? Will Nancy hold on to what seemed to her an all-giving mother with iron clutches and develop an everlasting hatred for her because of the frustration this mother is bound to inflict upon her? Will Charlie hold on to his masculinity with determination and strength throughout periods of passive withdrawal? Will Glenda be inclined to incorporate and project in quick succession and Nancy tend to incorporate persistently? Will Charlie be able to relinquish his œdipal attachment to his mother quickly to transfer it to someone more suitable to him in temperament? Will he merely withdraw without much hard feeling or will he progressively turn to his more placid father, creating a united front with him against the rest of the family? Maybe we shall find out; maybe not.'

ANALYSIS OF PREDICTIONS MADE IN THE PRELIMINARY REPORT

The questions asked concerning the future of the three children can be classified as intuitive predictions (4). They differ in focus: some refer to drive specific wishes, others to defense mechanisms, and still others to object relationships. The clearest prediction concerned the children's temperament. Glenda was expected to become a person who habitually alternates between initiative and giving up. Nancy was expected to become rigid and clutching. Charlie was expected to become a placid individual who would be capable of holding on with strength and determination. These predictions were based on the assumption that the children's preferred motor rhythms would be discernible in their future activities.

By implication, the children's preferred motor rhythms were correlated with specific zonal modes of drive discharge. The prediction of penis envy and of incorporation and projection implied that Glenda's dominant motor rhythms were appropriate for phallic and oral forms of discharge. The emphasis on clutching and on persistent incorporation suggested that Nancy's habitual motor rhythms were representative of oral-sadistic trends. The possibility that Charlie would hold on to his masculinity with determination throughout periods of passive withdrawal indicated the proneness to conflict which was predicted for him. Charlie's favored motor rhythm apparently suggested a propensity for anality but his response to his mother's stimulation was taken as an indicator that phallic trends would vie with the dominant anal drive organization.

The behavior of the children from infancy through latency was used to test the validity of the following intuitive predictions which were suggested in various ways in the preliminary report. The congenitally preferred rhythms of motor discharge would be discernible in whole or in part, with or without modification, in the children's motility and actions. The preferred motor rhythms of early infancy would be modified by maturation as well as by interaction with maternal motor patterns. Features of the preferred rhythms of discharge which were enhanced by the environment would not only become discernible in the children's temperament, but would decidedly influence their character formation, normal or deviant. Clashes between the child's and the mother's preferred rhythms of motor discharge would lead to specific conflicts and corresponding pathology. The preferred rhythms of motor discharge would prove to be representative of specific forms of drive discharge: phallic and oral in Glenda, oral-sadistic in Nancy, and anal in Charlie.

These predilections would lead to the following personality traits:

Glenda's propensity for sequences of phallic and oral discharge forms would lead to: 1, strong penis envy; 2, a temperament in which giving up for a very short time would alternate with reinitiating activities; 3, quick alternation between incorporation and projection.

Nancy's 'oral-sadistic' rhythm of discharge, if those about her continued to encourage tonic holding, would lead to: 1, unusual rigidity (perhaps of ego and superego); 2, ambivalent clutching and a hateful relationship to her mother.

Charlie's innate rhythms (gradual steady increase of tension to great intensities, maintained on a plateau and followed by a gradual descent), possibly suggestive of an anal form of discharge, together with his early ability to respond increasingly promptly to his mother, would lead to: 1, a temperament characterized by placidity, determination, and strength, unhampered by periods of withdrawal; 2, proneness to conflict and premature ego development; 3, a quick giving up of his œdipal attachment to his mother and a turning toward his father.[5]

FOLLOW-UP REPORT OF THE THREE CHILDREN

Glenda, even in the neonatal period, displayed a tendency toward sudden rises to high tension, and sudden abatement of it.

[5] It is interesting to note Dr. Escalona's remarks to the children when they were fourteen months old. To Glenda she said that she need not do the suggested task right away, she might come back to it later. To Charlie, she said encouragingly that he could do what was asked of him in his own way. Nancy, who could not relinquish test objects, was told that she could let go of the test items so that she might turn to a new thing offered to her.

After a short 'rest' she would abruptly resume her activity. (See Illustrations 2 and 3.) Glenda has continued to favor this rhythm of motor discharge over others. It is very likely that this particular rhythm is expressive of phallic discharge modus. Whenever Glenda's interest betrays an intense phallic preoccupation, her originally preferred rhythm of motor discharge becomes more intensified than is usually the case.

Before Glenda was one year old, her 'rest periods' were frequently occupied by a motor activity which consisted of sharp reversals between small amounts of inhibited and free discharge of tension (see Illustration 3). Because of the deficiency in the early recording, it is not clear when this type of rhythm began to be noticeable. It may well have started in the beginning of the oral-sadistic phase. When Glenda's brother was born, she was four years old; she became preoccupied with fantasies of biting and fears of being bitten and eaten. At that time the rhythm of her 'rest periods' could be seen to accompany her oral-sadistic strivings. A 'biting and chewing'-like rhythm was now clearly recognizable. It permeated most of her movement at that time and even overshadowed her usual phallic thrusts. Even though the oral tensions decreased in time, they left a permanent trace in Glenda's facial expression. Her perioral muscles became tense and her hitherto charming smile became forced.

As expected, Glenda has become tomboyish. Her behavior and her communications betray a strong phallic interest. This trend has been supported by her particular family constellation. But maturation and training widened Glenda's repertoire of rhythms. In the anal phase of development she learned to inhibit the free flow of her movement and she began to use a more gradual rise and fall of tension when necessary. Her mother had been able to tolerate the rapid rise and fall of tension in early infancy, but problems of bowel training intensified her own propensity for a more steady and more gradual mode of functioning. Glenda's mother was always able to maintain her excitement longer than her daughter. She was worried by Glenda's lack of enthusiasm for the pottie and pressed her to remain seated on it for a longer time than Glenda's inclination allowed for. A similar conflict arose later when Glenda found it difficult to sit still while doing her school work.

In the phallic phase, Glenda's preferred rhythm of motor discharge reigned supreme. Her mother took pride in her motor feats but expressed her conflict by both admiring and scolding Glenda for being on the go all the time and playing like a boy. At the same time she encouraged femininity by showering Glenda with dolls. Once when Glenda excitedly told a story which revealed sex play with a male playmate, her prevailing motor rhythm exhibited a wavy quality, which may have been vaginal in nature.

Pressed by her own needs, by her mother, and by the exigencies of reality, Glenda has evolved two distinctly different ways of behaving. One, when engaged in work, she seems tense, awkward, and unhappy; the movements of her writing, her drawing, and of other activities involving small muscle coördination, retain an oral-sadistic type of rhythm. Two, as soon as the arduous task is over, and even more evident when she can escape her mother's watchful eyes, she reverts to sudden eruptions of high tension; she jumps up like a jack-in-the-box and joyfully pursues her originally preferred phallic rhythmicity. Her purposeful, adaptive movements in gross motor activity have become skilful and she exhibits qualities of movement that attest her talent for motor feats. She does not mind sedentary activities as long as they do not last too long. What makes her unhappy is that she is not allowed to jump up periodically while she studies. She seems to fall in the category of Ferenczi's motor types (14). Because her rest or work periods have been artificially extended beyond her endurance, Glenda does not function intellectually up to her capacity.

Even in the newborn nursery, Nancy evidenced a dysrhythmia difficult to classify but clearly suggestive of deviant development. Her excitation was prolonged and intense, but most of all it was unpredictable in its course. She would go from prolonged stiffness to limpness of short duration. The strange quality of her states of tension was often produced by a mixture of cramping and limpness which would be followed by fluctuations between high tension, rapidly rising, soon subsiding, or persisting for a long time, and explosive eruptions of free and diffuse tension discharge.

Nancy's tendency to rigidity and cramping was encouraged by her mother, who provided her with objects she could clutch. Even though at about nine months Nancy was given more opportunity to move about freely and release her spasmlike contractions, her motility continued to be strange as she now tended to alternate rigidity with an exaggerated release to the point of limpness. At that time I asked: 'Will Nancy hold on to her mother with iron clutches and develop an everlasting hatred for her?' This did not happen. Instead Nancy developed a rigid attachment to her sister, who became her nursemaid and constant companion. Her aggression was openly expressed in unpredictable hitting out at her siblings.

Toward the end of the first year of life Nancy's rigidity combined with waxy limpness reached the point of catalepsy during sleep. Thereafter Nancy went through several periods of apparent relaxation of tension and greater ease. When her mother's encouragement of holding and clutching diminished, she became more mobile and caught up with motor functions in which she had been retarded. As she followed her 'softer' sister around, she became more pliable. When she joined the outdoor life of a group of children at about two or three, her excessive muscular tension subsided still more.

It is difficult to evaluate how Nancy's quite early toilet training influenced her development. Neither is it easy to say what changes occurred during her phallic phase at four or five. During most of our visits at that time and later in latency, she would sit slumped in a chair, speaking only when spoken to. She would mouth, distort her lips into a snout, or pucker them, chewing real or imaginary objects. At the same time she would fiddle with her fingers, pulling and releasing, pressing, twisting, and picking, all in an aimless, contentless manner. She would snap out of this perseverative behavior to snatch something from her siblings or pull it away with tension rather than strength. Once she got hold of the desired object, she handled it in the same random style as she showed without it. Possessive and reluctant to give up anything, she would become still more tense while clutching an object, but she became limply compliant in the presence of her parents.

Only recently could I again see some signs of improvement which may or may not persist. During my last two visits, which occurred when Nancy was nine years and eight months old, the excessive mouthing was no longer a conspicuous feature of her behavior. The impression of violence she gave as an infant and at times as a toddler no longer existed. But her total behavior was still unpredictable and deviant. When she danced at my request, her movements were perseverative, automatic, and stereotyped. Even though she was failing in two subjects, she reported that her teacher thought her brilliant. Her learning is done by rote. How similar her thought processes have been and still are to her deviant motor patterns can be best exemplified by the manner in which Nancy at five or six, and even now at almost ten, would recount the story of Goldilocks and the Three Bears. According to Nancy, Goldilocks tasted the porridge of the big bear and found it too hot, then she sat down on the big bear's chair and that was too hot; then she lay down on the big bear's bed and that was too hot. When she was younger, she showed her native intelligence when asked why the bed was too hot. She would quickly answer that the bear lay on it so long that he made it hot. But now her powers of rationalization are hampered further by an immature form of 'repression'. At nine she thought for some time before she answered the question why the chair and bed were too hot. With a sheepish smile she then explained that the sun had shone on the bed of the big bear and made it hot.

Both the records of movement and Nancy's total behavior suggest the following constellation of deviant drives. She seems dominated by several conflicting rhythms of discharge. Oral repetitive suckinglike tensions and releases, oral-sadistic biting, grinding, and holding seem to vie with each other and with various anal, anal-sadistic, urethral, and phallic spurts which hardly ever develop in an undistorted rhythm that is clearly recognizable. Whereas the 'anal', 'urethral', and 'phallic' ways of discharge almost disappear in the avalanche of oral impulses, the various kinds of oral discharge exist side by side. They seem to compete with one another and do not produce a compromise. To function Nancy must give in to one or another of her divergent rhythms, especially when there is enough environmental pressure on her to facilitate a selection. The inborn need for rigid responses which seem to be part of an oral-sadistic discharge rhythm (rocking, tensing) was fostered by early training and has become the main source of Nancy's primitive defense mechanisms. Threatened with being overwhelmed by too many divergent impulses, she responds by perseveration, the only means she has to prevent disorganization. Her mother has little to offer to help stabilize her modes of discharge of tension, and still less can she help her control diffuse discharge.

Nancy's early dysrhythmia seems to have been indicative of a clash between various oral libidinal and aggressive modes of discharge.

Even in the nursery Charlie gave the impression of being an important citizen. He looked and felt like a heavy viscous mass. He could respond to stimuli by a gradual increase of attention which attained high levels of intensity and only gradually subsided. In nursing he became increasingly excited and noisy, reaching a plateau of high excitement which gradually abated. He would fall asleep gradually and sleep long. His awakening was equally gradual, as he proceeded from depth to lightness of

leep and on into several stages of awakening. Once he reached
a high level of excitement he was capable of more explosive
movements and of many more variations of level and quality of
tension than during the rise and abatement of his excitation.
He was both very responsive to stimuli and able to absorb them.
During the time of gradual increase of excitation he took in
visually and acoustically what was going on. When his mother
stimulated him, his excitement rose quicker than usual. When
he was undisturbed his movements evidenced a prematurely
deliberate quality, although his coördination was by no means
better than that of the other children. His transitions were
smoother, his sequences much less disjointed than is usual for
infants and young children.

His mother and his siblings were intense, energetic, and
quickly changing. It was when Charlie began to sit with the rest
of the family and had to respond actively to solid food as well
as many objects offered to him that he began to withdraw; he
would show a vacant stare that left him in a world of his own.
Eventually he gave up reaching for objects handed to him, and
occupied himself only with his bottle and parts of his own body
which 'came to him' in his very own mode of discharge. This
mode included not only the rhythm of discharge, but also the
spatial configuration of stimulus and response. Charlie seemed
to prefer to have objects presented in space so that he could
reach for them by moving forward or laterally. His mother
habitually fed him while standing, her body in half retreat
and only her head bent forward and down toward him. The
spoon approached him from above while his siblings piled
toys on his table, thrusting them on him and removing them out
of reach. He withdrew from the spoon by turning his head sideways. When the spoon was held in front of him long enough, he
did reach forward and his lips got hold of it. When toys were
presented to him and moved horizontally in front of him while
he was in a supine position, he still took his time before he
reached, but he could do so with greater ease by a forward and

lateral movement. When they were held too high, so that he had
to direct his gaze and arm upward to get them, he would not
even look at them. This does not mean that Charlie could not
move in all directions. He tended to choose his preferred directions over others when he also had to do new things or adopt a
mode of discharge that required a quicker and more fluctuating manipulation of tension than the one he naturally favored.

On realizing that she needed to adjust to Charlie's ways, his
mother began feeding him with greater patience. But after
some time she would slide back into her accustomed pattern of
quick changes and alert readiness for new actions. It was hard to
understand precisely the basic clash between Charlie and his
mother, especially as it became clear that Charlie had a varied
and rich repertoire of rhythms available to him. He seemed to
function well, using all kinds of rhythms provided they were
subordinated to his basic over-all rhythm of gradual rise and
abatement of excitement. Once he reached a high enough plateau of excitement, he could include all kinds of variations of
tension.

My prediction when Charlie was nine months old was that he
would hold to his masculinity with determination and strength
throughout periods of passive withdrawal, and would prove
able to relinquish his œdipal attachment to his mother quickly
so that he could transfer his allegiance to someone more suitable to him in temperament. Thus far this has proved false.
Charlie's capacity to respond to people intensely and steadily
tended to distort my objectivity. The wording of my prediction suggests that, because I believed that Charlie's natural inclinations must be respected and that his struggle was deserv-
ing of support, I sided with the child against his mother.

As a toddler Charlie conquered his mother's preference for
standing up; he insisted that she sit down and hold him on her
lap. The intensity of his desire and the ponderous fashion in
which he gave orders pleased and amused his mother. There
was an excited quality about their relation, already presaged by
the 'talks' they had when Charlie was only a few weeks old.

Even in infancy Charlie alternated between constipation and loose stools. The period of toilet training was prolonged and the bathroom became the focal point of Charlie's relation to his mother. She had to sit there with him and engage in conversation long after he was able to attend to his own toilet needs.

His phallic needs became most evident in the bathroom, where he would also go when his mother was using it. He had begun to call his penis a 'boy' and he insisted for more than a year that his sister and especially his mother had one, even though he was allowed to observe that he was mistaken. With further progress of the phallic stage he seemed to adjust better to his mother's and his siblings' prevailing agility; but his speech became increasingly sexualized and he began to stutter. The clash between what seemed 'anal' modes of movement and thought with those which served his phallic attachment to his mother resulted in a succession of cramplike holding and explosive outbursts when he wanted to interest his mother in what he had to say. His siblings reached her more quickly, but he could in effect hold her longer as she was forced to wait patiently until he managed to 'eliminate' his words. When speech training improved his stuttering, he developed a variety of tics. In time Charlie became competitive and played with children, but he soon began to prefer staying home with his mother to being outdoors with his friends and siblings.

Charlie's history is a near-decade of struggling to adjust to the needs of his mother and to bend her mode to his own. The compromise formation between his own preferred rhythm and other rhythms impinging upon him during different maturational stages, from within and from his family, has led to clearly neurotic disturbances in his latency period.

He suffers from severe disturbances of learning. In the first three grades he dawdled over his work and stared vacantly instead of finishing it. He became compulsive in his need for perfection, but his thought processes and movements decelerated so much that he failed to grasp and solve simple problems. Placed in a classroom with a progressive teacher he is now doing rather well. But when his mother asks him a question that requires thought, he gets caught in a situation similar to his early feeding of solids. She stands over him, forcing herself to be patient, but she is ready to retreat in expectation of his failure. Only her head bends down to him. Their bodies are close but their gaze is apart. He begins to stare into space and slows down to the point of immobility. Her waiting only accentuates his failure and her leading questions fall flat as Charlie at that point is not accessible to her. He can answer the same question when the observer, approaching him at eye level, gives him ample time to gather his thoughts and helps him to arrive at the solution of the problem step-by-step. When he comes up with the right answer, he is sure of himself, yet he blurts it out explosively in triumphant, hasty speech.

Clinical data tend to strengthen the observer's impression that Charlie's preferred rhythm of excitation and discharge is of an 'anal' variety. This preference seems to be so strong that it colors and subjugates all other maturational phases and environmental influences. Faced with many divergent stimuli at five to seven months, when he was burdened by an influx of oral-sadistic impulses which clashed with his native rhythm, he had his hands full trying to cope with conflicting tendencies in himself. He had to withdraw from outside stimulations by his mother and his siblings who introduced what seemed a 'phallic' type of rhythm to complicate further his already extended battle front. His relation with his mother became quite intense and most satisfactory during the anal stage of development when normally mothers tend to regress to their own level of anality. It reached an even higher intensity in the phallic phase when he satisfied his mother's needs by consistently endowing her with a phallus and presenting himself to her as her phallus. But at the height of phallic interests, during the most intense œdipal relation to his mother, his stuttering became severe.

In latency, an obsessive trend threatened to take over. Toward the end of his latency, when early prepuberty began to appear, Charlie's blinking, shaking, and tic betrayed the renewal of conflicts between divergent forms of motor impulses. These were based on the early clash between his mother's and his own preferred rhythms of discharge. They were also currently renewed by the disharmony between his mother's preferred adult patterns and his own matured motor qualities.

PREDICTION AND OUTCOME

The periodic observation of these three children from the neonatal through the latency period indicates a correlation between their preferred rhythms of motor discharge and their specific drive endowment. Certain features of their originally preferred rhythms are still in evidence today. A result of the study which had not been predicted is that two of the children (Glenda and Charlie) function better and enjoy doing things more if they are free to use their originally preferred rhythms. Modifications that occurred through maturation as well as through interaction with persons important to the children enhanced or diminished certain components of the originally observable rhythms, but they did not eradicate the children's preference for these motor patterns. A clash between Charlie's and his mother's favored motor rhythms, discernible in early infancy, did become a source of Charlie's neurosis.

While the general proposition that preferred motor rhythms would correspond to favored component drives proved to be correct for these three children, specific predictions about their personality traits, based on this assumption, had a varying outcome. Some could not be tested, others seemed correct, and still others were wrong.

Whether Glenda's phallic orientation is primarily due to her congenitally strong phallic drive cannot be established with certainty. There are indications that this trend has been supported by the family. Her mode of giving up after a short while and resuming activities again is now interwoven into a complex pattern of behavior. When left to her own devices she proceeds in this manner. When she has to do sedentary work she seems persistent enough but at great cost to herself. There is not sufficient evidence of a tendency to incorporate and project in quick succession. Neither is it possible on the basis of observations and reports to judge the structure of her superego. What emerges instead with great clarity is Glenda's skill and enjoyment of activities in which she is free to use 'phallic' motor discharge. The 'oral-sadistic' rhythm of motor discharge is preferred in sedentary occupations, which Glenda neither enjoys nor excels in.

Nancy's early dysrhythmia seems to have been produced by a variety of unfused oral libidinal and aggressive rhythms of discharge. They often operate all at once, competing with each other and not allowing compromises with other forms of discharge. Until recently Nancy has continued to be very rigid and clutching. Her immature defensive structure seems to be based on rigid perseveration. Little can be said about her superego. We can say, however, that whereas Glenda has become a mildly neurotic child, Nancy remains highly deviant, possibly psychotic. There is some indication that she tends to incorporate persistently. The dearth of information about her behavior and her interests attests to the fact that her individuality can be best described as having 'form without content'.

Charlie's neurotic development can be traced since early infancy. His predominant rhythm since birth has been gradual ascent of tension from low to high levels, followed by a plateau of tension from which it gradually descends. This type of rhythm seems to correspond to one variety of discharge of anal drives (see Illustration 5). His mother tended to use abrupt rises of tension and was prone to many more fluctuations of tension than Charlie. The superimposition of this quality of her rhythm upon Charlie's own gradual and steady mode has led to early clashes between them. It has contributed significantly to Charlie's neurotic symptoms and traits. He has remained determined and placid but in his symptoms one can detect a vying between a gradual and an explosive ascent of tension. He did not give up his strong attachment to his mother, and there is no evidence that he turned to his father. His premature ego development may have fostered his neurotic solutions, and these in turn resulted in a restriction of the ego. It has remained clear throughout his development that he functions better when allowed to proceed in accordance with his congenitally preferred anal rhythm of discharge.

COMMENTS

The method of rhythm notation which was developed during a near decade of study was not used in the beginning of the observation of these three children. Descriptive recording does not do justice to the variety and combinations of rhythms observable even in the neonate. The classification of motor rhythms into 'oral', 'anal', and 'phallic' constitutes only a beginning of the study on correlations between motor rhythms and drive discharge. It is possible that only a few children show as pronounced permanent preferences for certain rhythms as could be seen in this pilot study. (Compare the views of Escalona and Heider [12].) It seems likely that a notation of motor rhythms will permit the detection of preferences for certain combinations of rhythms which may be representative of drive constellations. A comparison of motor rhythms with rhythms of autonomic responses (heart rate, blood pressure, respiration, etc.) would be helpful in examining the possibility that there is a central regulation of rhythms specific to processes of discharge of particular component drives, as hinted by Freud and Breuer (18). Rhythms of discharge through various channels need to be correlated with rhythms of stimuli which, according to Freud, may explain the physiological substrate of affects (21). Within the narrow confines of my study, I could only record early and later motor patterns which emerged with the progressive differentiation of id and ego.

As the rhythmicity of movement observable in these young infants became modified and incorporated into more complex patterns, the recording of rhythms alone did not suffice for the study of the role of motility in the children's development. As the ego took over the controls of motility, the original rhythms were altered by regulatory mechanisms ranging from primitive inhibition to adaptive controls which related to space, gravity, and time. Moreover, the shaping of movement went through different developmental stages that reflected changing relationship to objects. Further papers, based on the same pilot study, will consider how the ego regulates motility and adapts it to communicative expression (32).

CONCLUSION

Observation of three children from birth to about ten years of age suggests several areas for study in a larger number of subjects.

1. Preferences for certain rhythms of movement in early infancy.

2. Maturational and environmental influences that modify the originally preferred rhythms.

3. Early manifestations of disturbed development due to clashes between the rhythms of infant and mother.

4. Later behavior which may be derived from motor rhythms.

5. Identification of specific motor rhythms as expressive of specific drives such as oral, anal, phallic, and others.

6. Transitions between drive and ego dependent motility.

7. Methods of notation that would permit objective differentiation between rhythmic discharge of tension and the more mature components of movement which serve complex ego functions.

REFERENCES

1. BALLY, GUSTAV: *Die Frühkindliche Motorik im Vergleich mit der Motorik der Tiere.* Imago, XIX, 1933, pp. 339-366.

2. BARTENIEFF, I.: *Effort Observation and Effort Assessment in Rehabilitation* (Lecture at the National Notation Conference). New York: Dance Notation Bureau, 1962.

3. ———: and VENABLE, L.: *Laban Notation. A System of Recording and Studying Movement and the Application of Effort Notation in Rehabilitation.*

(Lecture at the Center for Cognitive Studies, Harvard University, 1963). Unpublished.

4. BENJAMIN, JOHN D.: Prediction and Psychopathologic Theory. In: *Dynamic Psychopathology in Childhood*. Edited by Lucie Jessner and Eleanor Pavenstedt. New York: Grune & Stratton, Inc., 1959, pp. 6-77.

5. BIRDWHISTELL, R. L.: *Introduction to Kinesics*. Louisville: Univ. of Louisville Press, 1952.

6. DEUTSCH, FELIX: *Analysis of Postural Behavior*. This QUARTERLY, XVI, 1947, pp. 195-213.

7. ———: *Thus Speaks the Body. I. An Analysis of Postural Behavior*. Trans. New York Acad. Science, Series 2, XII, No. 2, 1949.

8. ———: *Analytic Posturology*. This QUARTERLY, XXI, 1952, pp. 196-214.

9. ———: *Correlations of Verbal and Nonverbal Communications in Interviews Elicited by the Associative Anamnesis*. Psychosomatic Med., XXI, 1959, pp. 123-130.

10. ERIKSON, ERIK H.: *Childhood and Society*. New York: W. W. Norton & Co., Inc., 1950.

11. ———: *Identity and the Life Cycle. Selected Papers*. New York: International Universities Press, Inc., 1959.

12. ESCALONA, SIBYLLE and HEIDER, G.: *Prediction and Outcome*. New York: Basic Books, Inc., 1959.

13. FERENCZI, SANDOR: Laughter. In: *Problems and Methods of Psychoanalysis, Vol. III*. New York: Basic Books, Inc., 1955, pp. 177-182.

14. ———: Thinking and Muscle Innervation. In: *The Theory and Technique of Psychoanalysis. Selected Papers, Vol. II*. New York: Basic Books, Inc., 1952, pp. 230-232.

15. FREUD, ANNA: Problems of Infantile Neurosis. In: *The Psychoanalytic Study of the Child, Vol. IX*. New York: International Universities Press, Inc., 1954, pp. 69-71.

16. ——— and BURLINGHAM, DOROTHY: *Young Children in War-Time*. London: Allen & Unwin, Ltd., 1942.

17. ———: *War and Children*. New York: International Universities Press, Inc., 1944.

18. FREUD and BREUER, JOSEF: *Studies on Hysteria* (1893-1895). Standard Edition, II.

19. FREUD: *Three Essays on the Theory of Sexuality* (1901-1905). Standard Edition, VII.

20. ———: *The Ego and the Id* (1923). Standard Edition, XIX.

21. ———: *The Economic Problem of Masochism* (1924). Standard Edition, XIX.

22. ———: *Inhibitions, Symptoms and Anxiety* (1925). Standard Edition, XX.

23. FRIES, MARGARET: *Interrelationship to Physical, Mental, and Emotional Life of a Child from Birth to Four Years of Age*. Amer. J. Disturbed Child, XLIX, 1935, pp. 1546-1563.

24. ——— and WOOLF, PAUL: The Child's Ego Development and the Training of Adults in His Environment. In: *The Psychoanalytic Study of the*

Child, Vol. II. New York: International Universities Press, Inc., 1946, pp. 85-112.

25. ———: Some Hypotheses on the Role of the Congenital Activity Type in Personality and Development. In: *The Psychoanalytic Study of the Child, Vol. XIII.* New York: International Universities Press, Inc., 1958, pp. 48-64.

26. GLOVER, EDWARD: Quoted in Ref. 33.

27. GREENACRE, PHYLLIS: Problems of Infantile Neurosis. In: *The Psychoanalytic Study of the Child, Vol. IX.* New York: International Universities Press, Inc., 1954, pp. 18-24.

28. HARTMANN, HEINZ: *Ego Psychology and the Problem of Adaptation.* New York: International Universities Press, Inc., 1958.

29. JACOBSON, EDITH: *The Speed Pace in Psychic Discharge Processes and Its Influence on the Pleasure-Unpleasure Qualities of Affect.* Bull. Amer. Psa. Assn., VIII, 1952, pp. 235-236.

30. KESTENBERG, JUDITH S.: *Note on Ego Development.* Int. J. Psa., XXXIV, 1953, pp. 1-12.

31. ———: *History of an 'Autistic' Child.* J. Child Psychiatry, III, 1935, pp. 5-52.

32. ———: *The Role of Movement Patterns in Development. II. Flow of Movement and Effort. III. Shape, Flow and Shape.* In preparation.

33. KRIS, ERNST: *Laughter as an Expressive Process.* Int. J. Psa., XXI, 1940, pp. 314-341.

34. LABAN, R. and LAWRENCE, F. C.: *Effort.* London: MacDonald & Evans, 1947.

35. LABAN, R.: *Modern Educational Dance.* London: MacDonald & Evans, 1948.

36. LAMB, W.: *Correspondence Course in Movement Assessment* (1961). Unpublished.

37. ———: *A Method of Observation and Analysis of Physical Movement for Aptitude Assessment.* Unpublished.

38. MITTELMAN, BELA: Motility in Infants, Children and Adults. In: *The Psychoanalytic Study of the Child, Vol. IX.* New York: International Universities Press, Inc., 1954, pp. 142-177.

39. ———: Motility in the Therapy of Children and Adults. In: *The Psychoanalytic Study of the Child, Vol. XII.* New York: International Universities Press, Inc., 1957, pp. 284-319.

40. PIAGET, JEAN: *Les trois structures fondamentales de la vie psychique: rythme, régulation et groupement.* Schweiz. z. Psychol., I, 1942, pp. 9-21.

41. SANDER, L. W.: *Issues in Early Mother-Child Interaction.* J. Child Psychiatry, I, 1962, pp. 141-166.

42. SPITZ, RENÉ A.: *No and Yes.* New York: International Universities Press, Inc., 1957.

43. WOLF, K.: Observation of Individual Tendencies in the Second Year of Life. In: *Problems of Infancy and Childhood.* Edited by M. J. E. Senn. New York: Josiah Macy, Jr. Foundation, 1953, pp. 121-140.

44. WOLFF, P.: *Observations of Newborn Infants.* Psychosomatic Med., XXI, 1959, pp. 110-118.

THE ROLE OF MOVEMENT PATTERNS IN DEVELOPMENT

II. FLOW OF TENSION AND EFFORT

BY JUDITH S. KESTENBERG, M.D. (NEW YORK)

In the earliest postnatal stage it is difficult to disentangle the nuclei of functions that will later serve the ego from those we attribute to the id. Also, it is often hard to decide what part of it could already be described in terms of mental functioning. . . . It is clear that there is no ego in the sense we use the term for later stages; what the state of the id is at that level is unknown.

— HEINZ HARTMANN (*19*, p. 166)

As psychic functioning emerges and develops, motor apparatus available at birth as well as those maturing later are put into the service of drive discharge, the taming of drives, and adaptation to reality (*9, 12, 14, 15, 16, 18, 19, 27, 40, 41, 49, 50*). The newborn has at his disposal only primitive methods of regulation which do not permit satisfaction of his needs. His needs cannot be gratified nor wishes fulfilled without the help of his mother's ego, which organizes and tames the drives. The mother lends the child her regulatory apparatus and so prepares him for a more refined use of motility. Only when he has learned to control his body independently of his mother can he begin to adapt to the exigencies of reality.

Motor apparatus for taming of drives have a greater affinity to the ego than those serving discharge of drives. Mechanisms

From the Department of Psychiatry, Division of Psychoanalytic Education, State University of New York, Downstate Medical Center, Brooklyn, New York, and from the Long Island Jewish Hospital, New Hyde Park, New York.

I am grateful to Drs. Isidor Bernstein, Maurice Friend, Margaret Fries, Merton Gill, Heinz Hartmann, Edith Jacobson, Samuel Karlitz, Charles I. Kaufman, Ernst Kris, Samuel Lehrman, and others whose advice and helpful suggestions furthered this study. Drs. Hershey Marcus and Esther Robbins have made my observations more acute by their critical evaluation of my methods.

used in regulation of motility organize drive discharge. They are widely used by the ego in the sphere of its secondary autonomy. Motor apparatus that mature later in development equip the individual for adaptive functioning so that his actions can influence his physical environment in a significant way.

The present paper is concerned with the transition from early rhythmic motor patterns, which are put in the service of drive discharge, to complex motility controlled by the ego. It describes in detail methods of regulation that lay the foundation for adaptive motor functioning in adulthood. It introduces new concepts, partially derived from Laban's movement theory (34, 35), and an attempt is made to correlate these concepts with psychoanalytic formulations about the development of psychic structure.[1]

PSYCHOANALYTIC CONTRIBUTIONS TO THE UNDERSTANDING OF MOTOR PATTERNS

Freud's interest in rhythm ranged from the rhythm of excitation in the nervous system, rhythmic discharge of drive energy, the relation of specific rhythms of stimulation to qualities of pleasure and unpleasure, to the development of our concept of time from the rhythm of successive quanta of cathexis issuing from the ego (7, 8, 9, 10, 11, 13). Rhythm is a characteristic of all living tissue and Freud looked for its role in the lowest and highest modes of functioning.

Staerke (47, 48) suggested that the sensing and perceiving of our environment is mediated by kinesthetic awareness of the smallest movements which bring the outside world into the ego. He traced sensorimotor development in ontogeny and phylogeny and divided it into stages: one or more tonic stages, followed by a stage of interrupted tonus, which he subdivided into varieties of repetition—epileptic, rhythmic, reactive, and

---

[1] The introduction of new concepts necessitates new classifications and new terminology. A glossary, appended to this paper, contains explanations of new movement terms, as well as definitions of familiar terms which may lend themselves to misinterpretations.

delayed. He regarded tonic discharge as a rhythm with so extremely high a frequency that it is perceived as continuous. Hollos (22) believed that all of Staerke's sensorimotor stages pertain to forms of rhythm and agreed with his view that the highest forms of motility patterns are those with the lowest frequency of rhythm.

Spitz (46) pointed out that the joy and interest in repetition we see in young children wanes when they reach latency. He expanded Freud's view that rhythmic discharge in nonerogenous parts of the body can be sexual in nature, and suggested that rhythms are as specific as are zones for particular component drives. He concluded that the latency child is bored by repetition because he defensively shuns pregenital and genital temptations. Yet in a recent paper, Kaplan (24) reports her observations of joyful rhythmic games in latency. Both Spitz and Kaplan are right, however. Latency children begin to look down on rhythmic repetitions that are suitable for a specific drive discharge; they enjoy and seek games that regulate old rhythms by standards of skill and achievement. As Jacobson expressed so well, the developmental changes in pleasure and unpleasure depend on 'maturation of the ego which creates innumerable new channels for pleasurable functional motor and affective discharge' (23). Staerke postulated a developmental principle in phylogeny and ontogeny, namely: as development progresses the frequency of repetition decreases. Concurrently we can observe an increase in the variety and complexity of motor patterns. Kris (33) described the developmental enrichment of motor behavior as 'a transformation of rhythmical, automatic motor discharge into melody' in movement.[2] He suggested that we might understand ego development by studying the

---

[2] This does not mean that when movement acquires the pattern of melody it loses its rhythmic quality. In fact both rhythm and melody operate simultaneously. Ruckmick writes: 'In music the melody may be considered as a pattern of two dimensions, pitch and time. The chord adds the third dimension of depth of tonal mass or musical volume while rhythm provides the repeated periodic accent which adds movement to the whole' (42). Most definitions of melody refer to it as an organized succession of single tones.

development of motility, an inspiring proposal that poses two basic difficulties. Because of the global way most of us experience rhythm we tend to confuse the organ systems in which we perceive it and fail to analyze its components. Where a great many rhythms operate at the same time, some of them metrical, some ametrical, some simple, some complicated, we find it easier to experience the effects of continuity or discontinuity than to analyze all the variables.[3] Although we know that our feelings and concepts are derived in some way from kinesthetic perceptions, we cannot clearly see how this occurs (4, 22, 43, 44, 47, 48). The difficulty increases when we investigate comflex ego functions such as the sense of time and space. Here we are dealing with concepts partially derived from complex kinesthetic perceptions of various elements of movement.

Freud (8, 10) suggested that we perceive time as continuity by elaborating our perception of 'rapid firings of small quanta of cathexis'. But Bonaparte (2) was not convinced that 'our perceptions of space and time are originally and essentially an internal affair'. She believed that they 'must bear some relation to the fundamental reality of the universe . . .'. Freud's construct may have been derived from his kinesthetic perception of the most minute changes in muscle tension. Bonaparte, on the other hand, was impressed by feelings evolved from kinesthetic perceptions of movement elements which pertain to the

[3] Ruckmick defines rhythm in whatever sensory field it occurs as 'the perception of a temporal form or pattern in which individual members repeated periodically are consistently varied in any one or more of their qualitative and quantitative attributes' (42). I believe it would be more all-inclusive to say that the variation in biological rhythms is more or less consistent. Mosonyi (37) remarks that rhythm in general refers to the reappearance of periodic movement; in organic life it pertains to repetition of movement in response to stimuli. The repetition is essential; the periods, that is, the lengths of intervals between repetitions, are of secondary significance. Mosonyi, like most authors, thinks of rhythm as a repetition of movement after intervals of immobility with the implication that movement itself, regardless of its changing qualities, is the element of rhythm. My first notations and diagrammatic representations of movements were in part based on observations of two simple elements: movement and pause (30). For the definition of rhythm used in this paper, see the glossary.

'fundamental realities of the universe . . .', namely, space, gravity, and time. Laban's *(34, 35)* distinction between 'flow' and 'effort' brings into focus the feeling of continuity we experience while moving ('an internal affair'), as contrasted with our attitudes toward space, gravity, and time, the external forces to which we adjust in our psychomotor behavior.

The division of movement into elements of 'flow' and 'effort' may contribute to the clarification of problems posed by investigators of our sense of time and space. We have taken for granted that primary process thinking is devoid of realistic appraisal of space, gravity, and time, as exemplified in timeless and space-less flying in dreams. However, with the notable exceptions of Piaget *(38)* and Schilder *(44)*, little attention has been paid to our sense of weight and our relation to gravity. Spielrein *(45)* linked space, causality, and time as a triad and tried to trace the development of these concepts in children. Causal thinking is not only intimately connected with our attitude toward time and space, but also gravity. In contrast, primary process thinking is derived in part from the noncognitive perception of rhythmic changes in the flow of muscle tension. The regulation of tension flow which enables us to distinguish between continuity and discontinuity is one of the first steps in the development of motility control. Only after we have achieved mastery over the initiation, continuity, and stoppage of movement can we begin to time our actions in accordance with the exigencies of external reality.

RHYTHMS OF TENSION FLOW

Flow of tension refers to the relation between contractions of agonistic and antagonistic muscles. It is this relation that determines whether a particular part of the body is immobile, rigid, or relaxed; whether movement begins, continues, becomes intermittent, or ceases. At rest there is a balance between agonists and antagonists, a balance not static but rather consisting of minute swings from a hypothetical line of complete equilibrium. Movement is initiated by an imbalance between agonists and antagonists. The more the antagonistic muscles participate in the movement, the more they counteract and inhibit the movement. We then feel or see *inhibited or bound flow*. The less the simultaneous contraction of the antagonistic muscles, the less inhibited the movement. We then see and feel *free flow*. Various degrees of intensity can be observed in free and bound flow. The degree of intensity in bound flow is determined by the degree to which agonistic and antagonistic muscles oppose each other. The degree of intensity in free flow is determined by the degree to which agonistic muscle groups are freed from inhibition imposed by their antagonists. Extremely bound flow leads to rigid immobilization or cramping. Extremely free flow ends in immobilizing tremor. A high degree of free flow leads to the overshooting in movement so characteristic of young children (spilling, falling, running into objects).

The relation between flow and affect is best demonstrated by the fact that movements with free flow make one feel carefree, while movements with bound flow evoke that shade of anxiety that we call caution. Conversely, when we feel carefree we move freely, whereas caution makes us bound. Movements that maintain an even intensity in free flow convey steady confidence; in bound flow they give the impression of steady concern. Variations in levels of intensity may give a dreamy quality to our feelings; in free flow they are associated with pleasure, in bound flow with a sense of unreality. High degrees of intensity of free and bound flow evoke corresponding shades of feeling ranging from exuberance to depression. Low intensities of flow can be noted in manifestations of slight comfort and discomfort. Sudden eruptions of free flow are associated with surprise, of bound flow with fright. Gradual increase in freedom of flow is associated with feelings of pleasant expectation; gradual increase in bound flow can produce or express uneasy foreboding.

In the newborn, flow fluctuates widely and rapidly, but as the child grows older flow becomes more stabilized. Staerke described this trend as reduction in frequency of repetitions. It accounts for the fact that little children cannot sit still and that adults become increasingly sedentary. Within the range of normal temperamental differences we encounter vivacious people whose flow fluctuates more than it does in the average spontaneous person. Least fluctuation of flow occurs in phlegmatic and placid types and in solid, steady people who move with dignity.

Rhythms of flow of tension consist of more or less regular alternations between the elements of free and bound flow; there are also recurring changes in such attributes of flow as the degree of its intensity, the steepness of its ascent and descent, and the evenness of its level. Periodic alternations in the basic elements of flow and its attributes operate in the borderland between soma and psyche. The study of rhythms of tension flow seems particularly suitable for the exploration of the development of psychic functioning. But the immensity of the task that confronts us when we try to correlate early psychic processes with types of rhythmic motor discharge makes the path of investigation rugged and uncertain.

In the first part of this series (30), I presented a method of notation which helped me to correlate motor rhythms with specific forms of drive discharge, such as oral, anal, and phallic. From longitudinal observation of three children from the lying-in period to the age of eleven, I was able to develop this method further. At the start of the study I classified rhythms intuitively in accordance with clinical impressions derived from observation of total behavior. I was then most impressed by the individual tendencies to build up tension steeply or abruptly, to high or low intensity, to fluctuate in intensity or maintain long plateaus of even tension, to tend to relax, be rigid or limp in phases of immobility. These tendencies seemed to correspond to modes of drive discharge. In classifying motor rhythms as oral, anal, or phallic, I followed a long-standing tradition in psychoanalysis. Zone specific drives have been named after the somatic source from which they arose; terms of certain modes of complex ego functioning were derived from

their precursors in patterns of drive organization. Every eroto-
genic zone requires an optimum rhythm of discharge to insure
zone specific functioning; ego traits derived from zone specific
functioning are marked by attributes of zone specific rhythms;
for instance, stubbornness is an anal trait modeled after the
holding phase of the anal rhythm. It facilitates research to classify apparatus in accordance with the zone in which it operates
best and in keeping with the particular id-ego organization
into which it will become incorporated.

A diagrammatic presentation of typical rhythms of zonal discharge will serve to illustrate the manner in which these apparatus can be specifically defined in terms of elements and attributes of flow of tension. For clarity, I shall use quotation marks
when referring to 'oral', 'anal', or 'phallic' rhythms as apparatus
of motor discharge, and no quotation marks when referring to
oral, anal, and phallic drives or drive derivative activity.

In appraising the illustration one must keep in mind that
there are variations within the normal range of rhythms for
specific zonal discharge. What has been presented here is the
result of extrapolation from a number of observations and notations. Furthermore, one must keep in mind that it is easier to
observe sucking, biting, and chewing rhythms (Illustration 1,
I-a, I-b, I-c) than other zonal rhythms which are shrouded in
the privacy of the body. It is also important to note which
parts of the body involved in the zonal discharge have been observed. The sucking rhythms presented here refer to the changing flow in the labial and buccal muscles; the 'anal' rhythms
stem primarily from the recording of flow changes in accessory
muscles that contract simultaneously with the sphincter; the
defecatory rhythm is derived from changes in abdominal and
intercostal muscles; and the 'phallic' rhythms from observations
of manual and pelvic masturbation of young children and dogs.

With these qualifications in mind, let us examine the components of the rhythms shown in Illustration 1. Sucking rhythms
alternate between small intensities of free and bound flow (I-a).
Biting rhythms differ from sucking rhythms by the sharp rever-

Illustration 1

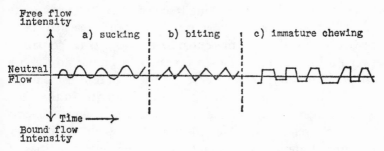

I) Oral rhythms

Free flow
intensity

a) sucking   b) biting   c) immature chewing

Neutral
Flow

Time ⟶

Bound flow
intensity

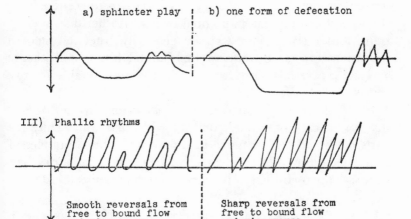

II) Anal rhythms

a) sphincter play   b) one form of defecation

III) Phallic rhythms

Smooth reversals from
free to bound flow
and vice versa

Sharp reversals from
free to bound flow
and vice versa

Diagrams of typical rhythms of tension flow that are appropriate for zonal discharge.

sals from free to bound flow (I-b). Short plateaus, in which the level of flow intensity is even, can be noticed in immature chewing (I-c). Later forms of chewing, not shown here, are characterized by alternations between steady and fluctuating levels; they can be noted when jaws begin to move laterally and the tongue participates in churning food.

'Anal' rhythms of tension flow often exhibit long plateaus

of evenly held flow of higher intensity, alternating with short phases of unevenness in lower intensities. Moreover, after a brief spurt of suddenly ascending free flow there follows a more gradual increase of bound flow until a plateau is reached (II-a). The defecatory rhythm presented here shows an alternation between a long plateau of high intensity in bound flow and a short phase of varying but lower intensity. It differs from the sphincter play rhythm not only in intensity but also in the steep ascent and descent and in the sharp reversals of flow elements (II-b). Both 'phallic' rhythms illustrated show alternations between small intensities of bound flow with high intensities of free flow; they are both characterized by a very steep ascent and descent of flow intensity. They differ in that the first is characterized by smooth transitions between ascent and descent of flow; the second exhibits sharp, pointed reversals rather than smooth transitions (III). It may well be generally true that smooth transitions are more frequent in libidinal forms of discharge and sharp reversals more frequent in rhythms suitable for discharge of aggression.

In the neonate we can record a great many rhythms of flow that follow each other and combine with each other. Different parts of the body may move in different rhythms. Samples of actual recording of flow changes in newborn infants can best illustrate the usefulness of the classification presented here.[4]

---

[4] In preparing these charts, the observer is aided by his kinesthetic identification with the subject. Free hand drawing of curves of changes in tension flow is obviously open to large subjective error in estimating the neutral line and the degree of change. Self-observation and practice as well as comparison with tracings of other observers, are methods used to reduce errors.

One observer cannot take note of simultaneous flow changes in different parts of the body but the record should contain successive alternations of free and bound flow and their attributes in all parts of the body.

One does not merely note a preference for a certain rhythm; one determines the balance of rhythms used by the subject by computing the ratio of the frequency of their manifestation. For example, Glenda (Illustration 3, I) at the age of eleven had a ratio of 'oral', 'anal', and 'phallic' rhythms = 4: 1: 2. In scoring and computing separately the ratio between free and bound flow and the ratio of recorded attributes of flow (even or fluctuating levels of attained intensity; high or low intensity; steep or gradual ascent and descent) one gains insight into

Illustration 2

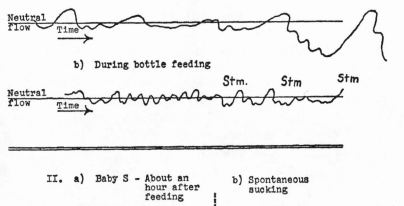

I. a) Baby C - Shortly after feeding

Neutral
flow   Time

b) During bottle feeding

Neutral
flow   Time   Stm.   Stm   Stm

II. a) Baby S - About an   b) Spontaneous
              hour after   sucking
              feeding

Neutral
flow   Time

I. Baby C (6 days old, birth weight 5 lb. 5 oz.)
   a) Sample of flow changes in movement of right hand, wrist and elbow.
   b) Sucking rhythm recorded from labial and buccal movement. Nurse helps
      by stimulating movements (Stm).
II. Baby S (4 days old, birth weight 8 lb. 10 oz.)
   a) Sample notation of flow changes in arm movements.
   b) Spontaneous sucking recorded from labial and buccal movement.

During nursing the oral rhythm, localized in the mouth, begins to approximate a metrical rhythm. Some time elapses before sucking is established in its pure form. Some babies must
be helped a great deal to make it regular (Illustration 2, I-b).
Congenital preferences for divergent rhythms interfere with

preferred methods of flow regulation. With this method one may discover that
a child in whom 'anal' rhythms are not particularly pronounced, still favors
even levels of bound flow because of his excessive use of certain 'oral-sadistic'
rhythms (Illustration 3, III). In extremely high frequency of 'oral-sadistic'
rhythms, bound flow may appear continuous rather than intermittent. The
comparison with records in various states of relaxation and tension, as after
and before feeding, helps us to decide what rhythm has been modified by the
interpolation of a prolonged plateau.

optimal functioning when they unduly intrude upon the oral rhythms and distort them. A baby's tendency to interpolate periods of bound flow, may cause him to cease sucking and to nibble on the nipple before he resumes feeding (2, I-b). Such a tendency is an attribute of 'oral-sadistic' rhythms and even more so of 'anal' rhythms (1, I-b and c, II-a and b). When a representative sample of recordings from various parts of the body indicates that 'anal' rhythms predominate over others, we suspect that the baby's congenital preference for such rhythms interferes with optimal sucking. The total record of Baby C, from which only a small fraction is reproduced here, indicated such a preference (1, II; 2, I-a and b).

A tendency to steepness of ascent of flow, may lead to gulping during feeding with a resulting overflow of milk (2, II-b). This tendency is an attribute of 'phallic' rhythms and of certain phases of 'anal-sadistic' rhythms (I and II-b). The sample of Baby S, presented here, exhibits a combination of 'oral', 'anal', and 'phallic' rhythms with the latter predominating. The relative dearth of sharp reversals from free to bound flow suggests a constellation of rhythms which will not favor aggressive discharge forms.

Drive endowment is closely correlated with congenital differences in apparatus of discharge. By classifying rhythms of tension flow in accordance with their suitability for specific zonal discharge, we may be able to assess their contribution to drive endowment. Changes in the ratio of rhythms in successive developmental phases may give us insight into the ways and means by which dominance of phase specific rhythms becomes established. Perhaps we may also get to understand better how the child's early methods of flow regulation become incorporated into the special modes he later 'chooses' for taming of drives and subordinating them to the aims of adaptive ego functioning.

To illustrate how congenitally preferred rhythms of tension flow, in interaction with maternal preferences for certain motor patterns, influence psychological development, I shall use examples from case histories of three children I have observed from the lying-in period through their latency *(30)*. Diagrams of these children's characteristic modes of rise and fall of tension, that could be observed in the newborn nursery, are reproduced here in the same form as the first two illustrations. Flow changes were actually written in this manner in later stages of the longitudinal observation of Glenda, Charlie, and Nancy.

Illustration 3

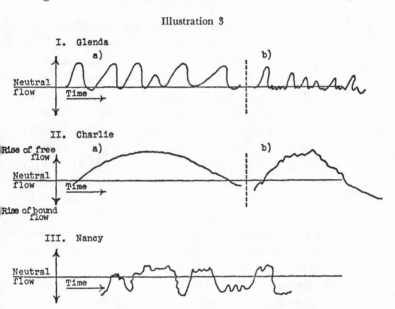

A schematic representation of preferred rhythms of tension flow in three children.

I-a) Glenda's 'phallic' rhythms of tension flow, preferred since the neonatal period until the present age of eleven and a half. Note alternations between high intensity in free flow and low intensity in bound flow, and prevalent steepness in ascent and descent of intensity.

I-b) 'Oral-sadistic' rhythms combined before the end of the first year into a sequence with 'phallic' rhythms (biphasic functioning).

II-a) Charlie's preferred rhythms have certain features in common with typical 'anal' and 'anal-sadistic' rhythms. (Gradual ascent to high intensity and prolonged evenness of flow.) Note the steeper ascent of intensity and the increase of fluctuations under stimulation (b).

III) Nancy's preferred 'oral-sadistic' rhythms mixed with other less identifiable rhythms. Note tendency to use bound flow, to sharp reversals, and the frequency of flow changes.

In the first paper of this series I tried to correlate the pre-ferred rhythms of these three children with my appraisal of their drive endowment from the observation of their behavior. The classification of these rhythms according to the elements of free and bound flow and their attributes (evenness of fluc-tuation of levels of intensity, high or low intensity, steep or gradual ascent or descent of intensity), helped me to define these children's predilections for certain modes of flow regula-tion. These predilections were characteristic of each infant and proved to be the *Anlage* for ego traits. A baby's preference for steep ascent of flow intensity that is quickly followed by a sud-den descent may predispose him for an approach to problem solving by transitory spurts of activity (3, I-a). A sequence of steeply ascending and descending free flow, followed by a quick alternation of small quantities of free and bound flow, may pre-dispose the child to biphasic functioning in which enthusiasm wanes quickly and is revived after a phase of repetitious labor-ing (3, I-b). A baby's preference for maintaining even levels of flow intensity, whether these appear chiefly in 'oral-sadistic', 'anal', or 'anal-sadistic' rhythms, may predispose him to stability, placidity, or attentiveness which are often already noticeable in early infancy. It may also lead to stubbornness, inflexibility, or other traits that cause clashing with the environment (3, II-a). A baby's preference for bound flow, especially if used to counter-act too frequent flow fluctuations, may cause the persistence of a primitive regulatory mechanism of freezing in immobilizing stiffness that promotes rigidity of defenses and retards ego de-velopment (3, III).

When these three children were eight months old I described their favored rhythms and correlated them with clinical ob-servations of behavior *(29, 30)*. At that time Greenacre *(17)* contrasted lolling and orgastic types of rhythm that could be observed in infants and emphasized that '. . . in fact, all lines of activity are present in some degree at birth or soon thereafter, but rise to a peak of maturational activity at different rates of speed. It is the maturational peak and its prominence in the

total activity of the individual organism which marks the phase.'
In full agreement with Greenacre's thesis I can say that all
rhythms of tension flow suitable for zonal drive discharge can
be noted in various parts of the neonate's body. The establishment of zone specific rhythmicity that is a prerequisite for drive
differentiation is contingent on the localization of specific
rhythms of tension flow in appropriate zones. Only then can
we speak of phases in which particular component drives gain
dominance.

In a paper read in 1945 (26), I contrasted the behavior of a
girl who masturbated to the point of orgasm since early infancy
with that of a deviant boy who rigidly immobilized his arms in
reaction to frustration (28). I spoke then of the persistence of
the original motor rhythms of the infant '. . . in a modified because higher organized form, throughout the life of the individual'. At the same time I stressed the importance of 'early organic
tensions and early organic reaction types' for the development
of individuality. Today I can be more specific: The newborn
infant shows preferences not only for particular rhythms of tension flow but also for particular modes of flow regulation. Intrinsic in each rhythm of tension flow is a type of flow regulation determined by the elements and attributes of that rhythm
(40). A preference for special forms of flow regulation may be
derived from various rhythms which have certain attributes in
common with each other. Rhythms become increasingly modified to conform to specific tasks; at the same time flow regulation becomes increasingly more complex. There is a hierarchic
ascendance in rhythm differentiation and in the refinement of
flow regulation, but the original preferences seem to persist
within the framework of higher organization.

FLOW REGULATION

Methods of flow regulation which help to organize motor discharge cover a wide range of mechanisms from neurophysiological apparatus, that decrease repetition and promote flow stabilization, to ego controlled modulation of flow intensity. Com-

plete stabilization of flow leads to immobility; partial stabilization confines flow changes to one zone of the body. Redistribution of flow elements and their attributes in different parts of the body operates in coördinated motor patterns.

Partial stabilization and patterned distribution of flow aid in the localization of zonal functioning. In successive stages of flow regulation the child gains a freedom of choice, limited to be sure, but allowing for a selection of elements of flow and their attributes in the service of a function. Fine gradation of intensities is a late acquisition that enables the child to modulate movement in the service of differentiated affective expressions and fine skills. Maturation of cortical connections enables the child to weave kinesthetic, touch, visual, and auditory perceptions into concepts of 'where, what, and when', and as he does he becomes progressively aware of space, weight, and time. Maturation of apparatus which seem designed for control of these forces of reality brings forth elements of 'effort' in our adaptive motor behavior *(1, 34, 35, 36, 43)*. 'Effort' elements operate in our approach to space directly or indirectly, to gravity by strength or lightness, and to time by acceleration or deceleration. Rhythms of flow of tension become subordinated to 'efforts' in the most advanced stages of flow regulation.

The motor patterns of neonates differ from each other in several ways: in the degree to which tension flow fluctuates *(14, 15)*, which forms the basis for their temperament; in the range of rhythms they exhibit from which we may assess their drive endowment *(30)*; in the preferences for certain attributes of flow from which we may be able to predict future preferences for dealing with reality through 'efforts'; in the methods of flow stabilization they favor in reaction to frustration *(5, 6, 14, 18, 26, 27, 28, 41, 49, 50)*; in the type of flow regulations they employ in the service of functions from which we may be able to predict their propensities for coping with their needs.

Stabilization of tension flow reduces the frequency of repetitions and counteracts rhythmicity. Within the normal range of flow fluctuations in neonates we encounter lively babies who may need a period of readjustment of flow before they settle down (3, I) and phlegmatic babies who look and feel heavy because their flow changes are few or develop too gradually to be easily noticed (3, II). So-called 'hyperactive' babies exhibit rapidly changing flow elements and their attributes (3, III). Some of them tend to use high quantities of free flow that lead to tremor; others can achieve stabilization only by immobilization through extremely high degrees of bound flow. Another rather extreme method of stabilization can be observed in limp immobility in which free flow decreases to a state of neutrality.

Immobilization through primitive methods of flow stabilization must be distinguished from immobility in relaxation and immobility in which we observe flow changes preparatory to movement. In relaxation moderate degrees of tension in agonistic and antagonistic muscles balance each other. Before movement begins, the parts of the body that will become involved in it exhibit changes in flow that enable us to predict whether movement will be initiated with free or bound flow. A redistribution of flow elements makes it possible to maintain bound flow in some parts of the body while others alternate between bound and free flow. The result of such a flow redistribution can be seen in neonates who maintain spontaneous rhythmic sucking of one hand by using the other hand to support it. In some infants who become attentive during defecation only those parts of the body which are involved in defecation undergo flow changes while the rest of the body maintains even flow as if in support of the discharge in the anal zone. In these instances flow redistribution led to a partial stabilization that was used to localize rhythmic discharge in one zone only.

A redistribution of flow elements that leads to a participation of all parts of the body in the main zonal rhythmic discharge can be seen in infants who become totally immersed in sucking. Fingers and toes follow the sucking rhythm and even those parts of the body which do not move, undergo flow changes in coördination with the sucking rhythm. A total involvement in a zonal discharge can be seen in infants who strain with their

LORETTE WILMOT LIBRARY
NAZARETH COLLEGE

whole body, grunt, and become red in the face during defecation. In those instances a redistribution of flow led to a centralization of rhythm in the service of a function. But centralization
of flow may also be achieved by successive rather than simultaneous changes of flow in all parts of the body. Rhythmic flow
changes may begin in a finger or a toe and spread through the
body before rhythmic discharge becomes localized in a specific
zone. Another form of centralization can be seen in infants who
maintain sucking during defecation or look around as they
nurse. They are able to integrate divergent rhythms with each
other into one central experience. When rhythms in various
parts of the body are not coördinated with each other, the observer gets the feeling that the baby is uncomfortable.

Despite the number of mechanisms available to the neonate
to aid him in localization of zone-specific functioning, his flow
regulation is rudimentary and undependable. He needs his
mother's flow regulation to maintain his. Holding the baby is by
no means a mechanical restraint of the baby; the mother employs sensitive mechanisms of flow regulation to re-enforce the
baby's own modes of regulation and to introduce new ones by
kinesthetic communication (3, 32).

Kris's suggestion that autoerotic sucking is an active repetition of the passive experience of sucking during nursing must
not be interpreted to mean that the child needs to learn the
sucking rhythm (33). The apparatus of sucking is available
even before birth. What the infant learns from the experience
of nursing is to maintain a continuity of sucking by actively re-
applying those methods of flow regulation that had been re-
enforced by the mother and mirroring those she had introduced.

Mothers enforce partial stabilization in the service of localization of zone specific rhythms in a number of ways: by picking up
a crying baby so that the mother's body creates a steady barrier
against flow fluctuations, in preparation for nursing (32); by
holding the baby firmly to prevent movements that interfere
with nursing; by positioning the baby in the crib in a manner
which facilitates hand-mouth contact; by blanketing the baby

securely to prevent interference from flow changes from the lower part of the body; by refraining from diapering or read-justing the baby who maintains stable flow during defecation or urination; and by holding or even lifting a child whose many flow fluctuations interfere with defecation.

Mothers encourage centralization in the service of localiza-tion of zone specific rhythm: by attuning their own flow changes with those of the baby they hold for nursing; by positioning him in the crib in a manner which allows for a spreading of the rhythm through the whole body (for instance, putting a baby whose rooting motions tend to culminate in hand sucking in a prone position); by limiting distractions which might strain the capacity of a child to absorb various stimuli into one central experience.

Localization of the appropriate rhythm in the appropriate zone is a necessary prerequisite for need satisfaction. It forms the basis for zone specific dominance and fosters drive differen-tiation. Disturbance of localization in infancy hinders the devel-opment of a cohesive ego organization. One of its early manifes-tations is an inhibition of autoerotic sucking that may hinder the orderly progression of ego functions.

Charlie, from birth, exhibited a dearth of flow fluctuations unusual for an infant (3, II). He felt heavy in one's arms be-cause he hardly adjusted his body to that of the person who carried him. Though heavy and phlegmatic, under special con-ditions Charlie learned a great deal by mirroring and later by imitation. Under stimulation he became more lively, and could function with all kinds of rhythms and with all parts of his body, provided he was allowed to build up tension gradually to a high plateau that he used as a base line for activity (3, II-b). Although he was disturbed by the many flow fluctuations of his vivacious mother and siblings, Charlie's vivid enjoyment of sucking persisted unabated. His ability to centralize helped him to maintain the continuity of sucking and to absorb many di-vergent stimuli into a whole experience (30). Charlie's mother regularly pulled his hand out of his mouth, admonishing him playfully to be a good boy. Possibly because of her own discomfort in holding the baby to whose rhythm of flow she could not adjust, she resorted to prop feeding relatively early. For this reason Charlie was not deprived of sucking. The fact that the bottle was left to him to do with as he pleased, allowed for a longer sucking experience than if he had been held by an impatient feeder. His talent for stabilization and centralization of flow kept him contented and in good contact with his environment. However, when he began to teethe, it became evident that an inhibition of hand-to-mouth movements had diminished his resources for soothing himself. He hardly rubbed his gums and would not hold a zwieback in his hand to feed himself.

A similar, but much more serious defect in the development of the executive functions of the ego could be seen in Nancy who exhibited an excess of flow fluctuations from birth. Nancy had very limited resources for flow stabilization. She tended to veer from extreme bound flow to limpness. In a prone position she would establish hand-mouth contact while rooting. But when sudden jerks of free flow or a sudden decrease of flow would disrupt the continuity of sucking, she responded with excitement that would soon lead to stiffening of the whole body. She would suck vigorously and continuously when her mother held her for feeding in the hospital. As soon as she came home she was left on her own for a greater part of the day. In addition her formula had not been changed so Nancy had to consume great quantities before her hunger was satisfied. She seemed to suck forever on the propped bottle and would not release the nipple even after the bottle was empty. Her frequent flow changes were held in check by a continuous maintenance of bound flow in her whole body, a method that insured uninterrupted holding on to the nipple. The immobilization of the body in the service of localization had the effect of isolating it from the oral experience. At the same time the tonic hold on the empty bottle enhanced libidinization (and aggressivization?) of the jaw muscles at the expense of the rest of her body. Nancy could neither suck her hand nor use it for reaching. Her hand as well as her other limbs became instruments of holding. She would clutch objects that were handed to her for a long time. As soon as she could stand she would remain in that position for very long periods of time, as her stiff spine, bound legs, and clutching hands prevented her from moving. She used tonic immobilization in the service of functions even where stabilization of flow became a hindrance rather than aid for functioning. It was interesting to note that Nancy could be soothed when she was crying by the very same quick and irregular fluctuations of tension flow which she had overcome by habituation to steady bound flow. Her mother would rock her with great abruptness and with a manner that impressed me at the time as both absent-minded and impatient. It seemed to me then that the mother's rocking could release Nancy's excessive boundness, as she was moved in a familiar way which became pleasurable when she was held securely.

Kinesthetic perceptions of rhythmic zonal discharge rarely gain access to consciousness. As they convey to the infant in which manner parts of the body are moving toward and away from each other, they become firmly embedded in their own creation—the body ego (4, 20, 21). In contrast to this, visual and acoustic perceptions seem designed to awaken consciousness and to make flow regulation subservient to psychic representations (9). All apparatus that promote consciousness tend to stabilize flow and to delay repetition.

Frequent flow changes reduce perceptivity for external stimuli and conversely, repetition of flow changes increases whenever apparatus serving perception of external stimuli cease functioning. In coma, the eyes usually move at irregular intervals, in varying intensities and in various rates of increase of free and bound flow. At times the rhythm becomes metrical and free flow changes into bound in a manner reminiscent of 'oral' rhythms (1, I-a). During awakening from coma, when seeking movements reappear, the spontaneous rhythm of eye movements interferes with attempts to follow objects until a state of consciousness is reached (25). Similar changes in eye movements reflect the changing states of drowsiness and alertness in the neonate (3, 52).

Even in states of alertness, neonates have little control over the flow of their eye movements. They can only be induced to follow visual stimuli when objects are moved at the same rate of speed, with the same gradually evolving flow of tension by which their eyes move spontaneously. We can deduce that the child is pursuing the object from the fact that he maintains the direction in which the object is moving much longer than he does without the visual stimulus. Visual pursuit not only effects localized delay of repetition but also stabilizes the flow in the rest of the body. When the newborn follows visual stimuli he becomes quiescent. Either his body becomes immobilized by partial stabilization of flow or all the body parts strain toward the stimulus in consonance with the movements of the eyes (centralization).[5]

In response to external stimuli, the rhythm of spontaneous movements becomes modified in conformance with the nature of the stimuli. The newborn reacts to the rhythmic flow of milk by a modification of his spontaneous rooting and sucking that brings out a pure 'oral' rhythm in the oral zone. At the same time partial stabilization of flow inhibits rooting movements in the rest of the body, or centralization of flow effects integration of flow changes in all parts of the body with the dominant 'oral' rhythm. In this manner a metrical 'oral' rhythm becomes localized in the oral zone and the continuity of sucking is preserved.

Flow regulation not only maintains the continuity of zone specific functioning, it also plays a role in the initiation or cessation of localized activities. Onetime rhythmic units are used as transitions to flow stabilization, in the beginning and at the end of zonal functioning. Free flow may effect the turning of the head away from the breast before the baby turns back to it and settles in a nursing position. Similarly, a baby may respond to a

---

[5] All data on neonatal eye movements presented here are based on my own observations. Some of them have been described in accounts of more systematic observations of the newborn (3, 39, 52).

moving object by first moving his eyes away from it and only then pursuit of the visual stimulus begins.[6] Transitions from rhythms of flow to flow stabilization that end motor discharge are seen when a baby uses bound flow to push out a nipple or tighten his lips and relaxes tongue or mouth in gradually decreasing free flow until he reaches the neutral flow of rest or peaceful sleep. When a baby tires of following objects, he may cease to respond, close his eyes, or blink. We see in these mechanisms of flow regulation a tendency to limit repetition not only to adapt to a stimulus but also to shut it out *(8, 18)*.

Some newborn babies are so entranced by looking or listening that they stop sucking; others close their eyes or stare ahead as if to protect themselves against disturbing visual stimuli. Hands get into the infant's line of vision as they move to the breast in preparation for fingering it during sucking. When the infant turns to the breast the hands begin to move by following the eyes but the eyes may also follow the hands. Visual pursuits become incorporated into the eye-hand-mouth system in phases preparatory for need satisfaction. By guiding the hand to the mouth and to objects, eye movements reduce flow fluctuations in the arm to conform to their own rhythm. When an excessive stabilization of flow in the eye muscles is used to shut out stimuli, the biphasic eye movements that prepare reaching are considerably reduced and the rhythm of hand movements remains unmodified. As a result too frequent changes in the flow of arms prevent neutralization of energy that is necessary for the establishment of the hand as the executive organ of the ego.

While in the hospital Nancy would follow objects with her eyes in the short phase when she was peaceful. She looked intently when her mother held her for nursing. At home she was

[6] Two interrelated rhythms are described here: 1, the alternation between free and bound flow, and 2, the alternations between centrifugal and centripetal movements which Lamb called the 'flow of shape' *(1, 31)*. Free flow initiates movements that veer from the midline; as the head or the eyes near the end positions, antagonistic muscles begin to contract in response to stretching of muscles and tendons, and bound flow breaks the lateral movement. For movement to continue, flow becomes free again and the direction of the movement reverses itself.

left in a darkened room with the bottle propped on her pillow. As her whole body became immobilized to support her hold on the nipple her hands would hardly get into the line of her constricted vision. Long after her contemporaries began to reach, Nancy would look at a rattle, listen to its noise, bring her head forward, open her mouth, but her 'bound' hands would not move to reach it. When she became more mobile she reverted to aimless mouthing and 'fiddling' with her hands and feet that retained the 'oral' and 'oral-sadistic' rhythms of her neonatal phase (3, III). She would look intently 'doing nothing, saying nothing', not only in her infancy but in later stages of development as well. Her steady looking was isolated from her manual and intellectual performance. When Nancy was fed solids she would clutch a spoon in each hand. This clutching continued after feeding very much the same way she held the nipple in her mouth after she finished sucking. The tonic holding retarded the development of biphasic actions such as reaching and grasping. When she finally did begin to reach she would grab the hand of the examiner rather than the object. It looked as if she perceived the hand as a holding instrument; when she released the grip she may have been reaching for the other person's hand to retrieve her 'lost instrument'.

When rigid immobility is used for partial stabilization of flow, the immobile parts of the body cease functioning. Once movement is released, numerous fluctuations of flow are brought about by the fact that rhythms from different parts of the body interfere with each other rather than modify each other. Each new function must be learned as a separate experience by a new process of localization in a new functional zone.

Nancy immobilized her hands during feeding and had to learn to reach as a separate experience, isolated from the restricted oral organization she had to adhere to.

Centralization in the service of a function uses all body parts simultaneously or successively; rhythms of flow arising in different parts of the body modify each other as they become integrated into a functional organization. When a zonal activity

ceases, the modified rhythms can be used in the service of other functioning. When a child's power of centralization is strained to the limit, he may need to withdraw from stimuli by a complete stabilization of flow in order to recuperate. He may also defensively restrict functioning to avoid disorganization.

Even as a newborn Charlie reacted to rhythmic acoustic stimuli with what seemed a high degree of attentiveness. Visual and acoustic stimuli tended to further reduce his already scanty flow fluctuations. During the first few weeks of life he was able to absorb visual, tactile, acoustic, and oral experiences all at once so that listening and looking became part of the early feeding situation even during prop-feeding.

Charlie's motor development was quite advanced: he grasped objects early and manipulated them with a purposiveness unusual for his age. He became selective in the rhythms of tension flow he used for different functions. But he often lapsed into a vacant stare that seemed to remove him from the world around him. The dazed staring seemed to shut out stimuli from inside and outside.

Charlie was not only prevented from autoerotic sucking but also from playing with solids. Objects were presented to him to distract him from messing and interfering with the mother's spoon feeding. At first Charlie was spellbound by objects and kept still during feeding, but he became dazed when objects were removed and substituted by others before he could finish his thorough examination of each toy. He would cry and refuse solids, but would be content drinking from his bottle in his crib. He would not hold the bottle or a zwieback and he stopped reaching for objects, but he did not immobilize his hands as Nancy did; he used them to play with his feet which no one could take away from him.

Charlie restricted functioning selectively to avoid displeasure. Even when he immobilized his hands, they did not cease to play a part in feeding or play. The flow changes preparatory to reaching could be observed in his resting arms. He did not isolate parts of his body from each other but he isolated his body totally or partially from contact with external stimuli that interfered with his preferred rhythm of tension flow (30).

Even in withdrawal he used centralization of flow in the service of the defensive shutting out of the world around him. The flow of his whole body adjusted to the far-away look in his face. In his crib he would come to life again. Undisturbed he would practice motor skills and evolve a great many modifications of rhythm which he could use for differentiated functioning. When he could engage in zonal activity without undue interference, he was able to apply the rhythms that had been modified when he learned something new. He would learn little when he could not use centralization in approaching problem solving, and he would learn instantly where the use of already familiar rhythms or their attributes were required. He would watch a psychologist keenly as his whole body was engaged in flow changes mirroring hers. When she finished the demonstration of a test item he immediately knew how to proceed although he was not capable of it before the demonstration. When he was much older and had learned to shun examinations in school, he responded poorly to verbal instructions and acted dazed. Even then he could learn with eagerness when one took special care to approach him gradually and to let him use his own methods of problem solving. Mechanisms of flow regulation that could be observed in Charlie's first year of life became incorporated into his executive and defensive ego functions.

The localization to appropriate zones of all zone-specific rhythms begins early in life (17). Methods of flow regulation that contribute to drive differentiation in stages that follow the oral are not only dependent on maturation of specific apparatus of control but also on all previous zonal experiences. Early methods of flow regulation extend to the anal and urethrogenital zones before zone-specific flow regulation can be established in these areas. For that reason none of the partial drives gains a dominance comparable to oral dominance. Throughout life more or less 'pure' oral rhythms can be seen in the flow of tension in facial movement, in purposeless motility of hands and even feet, as well as in many purposeful work movements that require frequent repetition.

At birth babies may show a predilection for rhythms suitable for anal or phallic discharge or for rhythm attributes that promote a flow regulation conducive to the differentiation of 'anal' (2, I) or 'phallic' rhythms (2, II). In those instances a modification of 'oral' rhythms by the divergent discharge occurs long before 'anal' or 'phallic' rhythms normally gain dominance. We then encounter precocious development while at the same time functions that depend on optimal 'oral' rhythms may suffer.

As rhythms become localized in appropriate zones the child begins to use them selectively in a pure form for drive discharge and in a modified form for neutralized discharge. Once a repertoire of modified rhythms of flow becomes available for adaptive functioning the child begins to use selection of rhythm attributes as a method of flow regulation. From the range of optimal combinations of rhythms and their attributes he will select those he likes best. To reach an object he may prefer to use even flow which will help him not to deviate from the shortest route to the object, or he may change his flow a number of times and stop himself in time with an excess of bound flow. To open a cabinet he may select high intensity of bound flow that develops gradually, or he may use a number of spurts of suddenly ascending free flow without resorting to high intensity in order to accomplish the task. Controlled selection of flow attributes in the service of functions are forerunners of 'efforts' which are elements of movement we use to make an impact on the environment (1, 34, 35, 36, 43). Subordination of flow changes to control through efforts is a highly advanced method of flow regulation that is not fully established until adulthood. Its development overlaps with a progressive refinement in selectivity that enables us to graduate flow intensities by modulation and to organize selected sequences of rhythmic units in phrasing. Highly differentiated selectivity in flow changes and subtlety in affective expressiveness are interdependent achievements. Flow of tension in graduated intensities evokes a succession of shades of feelings, and finely differentiated affects express themselves in shadings of flow intensity. A repeated sequence or 'theme' of graduated flow intensities gives 'melody' to movement. As Kris (33) suggested, melody of movement rates high in the developmental scale of ego functions. It may well be that it is the individual melody of movement that differentiates adult genital organization from its precursors in infancy.

At this stage of my study I am not able to give more than general data on the hierarchy of flow regulations. Nor am I able to say in which phase of maturity single 'effort' elements can be noted and when they become consistent psychomotor elements. But the following conclusions are possible. 1, The various rhythms of tension flow seen in the neonate become differentiated in such a way that pure rhythms serve localized drive discharge and modified rhythms are used in drive derivative functioning as apparatus of secondary autonomy. 2, Methods of flow regulation derive their style from the elements and attributes of rhythms from which they evolve. 3, Selectivity in flow becomes differentiated with progressive development of the ego's control over expression of affect. 4, Controlled selection of flow attributes is a precursor of effort. 5, Developmental trends overlap and interact in such a way that patterns of tension flow reflect changing constellations of drives, while patterns of effort subordinate the flow of tension to their adaptive aims and reflect transitory and permanent ego attitudes to the world in which we live.

DEVELOPMENT OF EFFORTS

The newborn infant is not capable of organized action and his motor behavior bears little relation to reality. He has at his disposal primitive regulatory mechanisms that he can use to stabilize flow and limit repetition. With his mother's help he develops means to localize zone-appropriate rhythms and to modify divergent rhythms in the service of functions. Even when he grows older, the child uses methods of flow regulation that are derived from the qualities of rhythms he most frequently experienced. Gradually he develops enough control over his own flow of tension to enable him to select optimum rhythms o

:onal discharge and those attributes of rhythms that are most uitable for the execution of a task. Throughout life he re- ains a preference for patterns of movement that evolved from hythms he enjoyed most. When maturation of apparatus for lynamic dealing with the forces of space, gravity, and time :nables the older child to change his environment through work ınd affective communication he still favors 'efforts' that have he greatest affinity to his originally preferred flow patterns.

Flow of tension initiates movement, maintains its continuity, ınd stops it. Without it, no 'effort' is possible. Although 'effort' :lements subdue and govern the flow of tension, they are genet- cally and currently dependent on it. 'Effort' elements in our novement reflect changes in our attitudes toward: (1) space,)y approaching it directly or indirectly; (2) gravity, by relat- ng to weight with strength or lightness; and (3) time, by ac- :elerating or decelerating the pace of our movements. 'Effort' s comparable to a rider who, in complete control of his horse, nay choose to take a direct or an indirect route, or to whip he horse with strength or lightly, or to speed the pace or slow t down—all this provided the horse has been tamed and trained o carry a rider, to start and stop, and to change the rhythm of ts gait in subordination to the rider's commands. To complete he metaphor, one may add that the trainer has acted in the louble capacity of training the horse and the rider as well.[7] 't is apparent from this metaphor that 'efforts' are those compo- ıents of movements by which the ego controls drives in the serv- ce of adaptation to reality (9). They are complex functions of

[7] Laban (35) depicts efforts as arising from the medium of 'flow of effort'. I ıave changed this term to 'flow of tension' to indicate that movement can ·roceed with flow independently of effort. I have used only a few of Laban's ːrms and only such definitions and modifications of his concepts as are neces- ıry to fit his movement theory and Lamb's contributions to it (1, 34, 35, 36, 43) ıto the framework of psychoanalytic psychology. I am indebted to Irma ³artenieff and Warren Lamb who taught me the principles of movement theory ınd effort notation, but they are in no way responsible for my method of rhythm ·otation nor my modifications and expansions of Laban's and Lamb's movement heories (30, 31).

the ego which reflect our feelings and our concepts of space weight, and time.

In stages of transition from adaptive flow regulation by selection of flow attributes to adaptive control through 'efforts', the observer is often in doubt whether he has seen a precursor of 'effort' or a mature 'effort' element. A toddler playing carpenter with his peg set seems to use strength or directness. But it may well be that he has merely selected flow attributes for his movement which have an affinity to these 'effort' elements. We can use several criteria to distinguish a forerunner of 'effort' and mature 'effort': first, we must ask ourselves whether that type of directness or strength could be used to make an impact on real objects. Can we interpret these motor patterns as expressive of a dynamic relationship to space or weight? Could they be used to convey a direct approach to problem solving or to communicate authority? Since we are dealing here with transitions to elements of 'effort' we may be uncertain in our answers. Once 'effort' elements are clearly established, trained observers will recognize them without doubt.

Aim-directed selection of flow qualities is prerequisite for dealing with reality through 'effort'. It is a part-function of 'effort' which becomes integrated with other components into the complex organization of 'effort' patterns. We can recognize the affinity of certain flow attributes to specific elements of 'effort' and may be able to predict future preferences for certain 'effort' elements from earlier preferences for the corresponding flow qualities.

1. There is an affinity between evenness of flow levels and a direct approach to space. In direct movements, we may utilize even flow to achieve steadiness, either in the entire action or in one phase of it. To become direct in our movement, we not only select sequences and attributes of tension flow that will give impetus and continuity to our action, but we direct our attention to one spatial plane in which we decided to proceed and restrict the use of other planes. We may use directness for the precise execution of a task, as driving a nail into a plank, or we may use

it to communicate a definite attitude, as 'hitting the nail on the head' or 'getting to the point'.

When a child selects even flow for his movement in order not to stray from his path, his attention is centered on restricting his flow fluctuations so that they do not interfere with his attempt to reach an object. Such an aim-directed control of tension flow is accomplished through taming of impulses to move every which way. It differs from earlier types of regulation by stabilization of flow, as it is specifically concerned with adjusting the body to function in space. It constitutes a stage in the development of mastery of space and as such is a forerunner of a direct approach to space through 'effort'.

2. There is an affinity between variations in levels of intensity of tension and an indirect approach to space. Uncontrolled variations of flow intensity may convey unsteadiness, absent-mindedness, or dreaminess. Deliberate changes in flow intensity that preserve the continuity of movement in winding from one spatial plane to another, indicate a flexibility that has to be attained before we can develop indirectness of approach. Indirect 'efforts' incorporate planned changes in flow intensity into actions which require the successive use of two or three planes. They are employed in tasks such as spinning wool or wringing a towel dry. They communicate modes of affect and thought in gestures when we 'spin a yarn' or 'wring a subject dry'.

3. There is an affinity between high intensity of tension flow and strength. High intensity of flow conveys strain or enthusiasm. Deliberate increase of flow intensity to accomplish a purpose is a precursor and component of organized actions in which we cope with weight. It reflects the degree of intent that motivates us to use strength as an 'effort' to oppose gravity. We apply strength when we lift weights, give orders with authority, and communicate our affective attitudes in such phrases as 'weighty considerations' or 'the gravity of the situation'.

4. There is an affinity between small quantities of tension flow and lightness. Through the use of small quantities of tension we may convey lack of concern, delicacy, or slight discom-

fort. Before we can approach objects with lightness, we must be able to decrease the intensity of tension flow at will. The 'effort' element of lightness incorporates diminutions in flow intensity into certain phases of actions that are based on previous success in overcoming gravity, and operate from a base of levity. We employ lightness in manipulating light objects, in dancing on tiptoes, and in gestures that express 'lightness of spirit' or an attitude of 'treating a matter lightly'.

5. There is an affinity between steepness of ascent or descent of flow and acceleration. Sudden changes in flow intensity merely connote quickness of response. A deliberate increase of the rate with which tension rises or falls is an achievement of a stage in the development of our sense of time. We use steep ascent of flow to start a movement in high speed and we use steep descent of flow to stop abruptly. We incorporate those flow changes that reflect our sense of urgency into actions in which we oppose the passage of time. We accelerate our speed in walking to get somewhere faster, and use acceleration for the communication of attitudes to time that language expresses in such phrases as 'beating time' or 'having no time'.

6. There is an affinity between gradual ascent and descent of flow, that gives the impression of leisure, and deceleration. We are able to select the degree to which we decrease the rate of ascent or descent of tension only when we begin to understand that flow changes progress in time. When a child begins to appreciate that dawdling can make him late, he may begin to use the appropriate rate of increase or decrease of tension flow to effect a slow start or a slow stopping of movement. The 'effort' element of deceleration incorporates gradual changes of flow intensity into actions, retarding the passage of time. We may decelerate the rate of our speed to conform to the speed of a machine we operate, or we may decelerate the speed with which we walk when we decide to get to an appointment on time instead of too early. Through deceleration we convey our affective attitudes to time that language expresses in phrases as 'having plenty of time' or 'being a sluggard'.

'Efforts' are patterns of movement that we employ in our dynamic adjustment to forces of reality. In physical work, through which we exercise our influence over our environment, we are required to use more 'effort' elements than in any other activity, with the exception of sports. People are suited for certain occupations when their individual preferences for specific 'effort' elements coincide with the 'effort' required in the work involved, but training habituates one to use all the elements of 'effort'. Rhythms used in sequences and combinations of 'effort' elements make work enjoyable rather than a chore *(36)*. Rhythms of tension flow mark the individuality of drive derivative work habits, such as 'oral' swaying to-and-fro or 'anal' straining and releasing (see Illustration 1, I and II). Elements of 'effort' by themselves can be used to compose a rhythm as can be seen in alternations between strong and light beats. The choice of work rhythms and rhythms in art reflects individual preferences for tension flow expressive of drives, as well as for sequences of 'efforts' that represent ego attitudes.

Not before adolescence do we acquire the ability to use three elements of 'effort' in one action. Preferred combinations of effort and flow elements in phrases of movement become permanent characteristics in adulthood. Elements of 'effort' and their combinations are interrelated with a wide range of qualities, from physical characteristics and style of movement to affective attitudes and modes of thinking. Which of these qualities will prevail in our use of 'effort' depends on the degree to which tension flow and psychic representations of space, weight, and time contribute to the relatively autonomous apparatus that makes 'effort' possible *(16, 41)*.

At the age of ten and a half, Nancy surprised me during two successive visits in which neither mouthing nor 'fiddling' was prominent. But notation of her rhythms of tension flow revealed that 'oral-sadistic' rhythms far exceeded any others in her repertoire of movement. Even though 'oral' rhythms are generally used more frequently than others, especially in hand and face movements, the ratio of 'oral': 'anal': 'phallic'

rhythms of 13:1:1 computed from Nancy's record deviated sub-
stantially from the average. Notation of 'effort' showed a preference for lightness and avoidance of strength. Nancy tackled
problems requiring strength by a controlled increase of bound
flow.

At eleven and a half Nancy was more productive and spontaneous than ever before. But her long-standing tendency to repeat could be noticed in her drawing of the inside of the body
which she filled almost completely with small dots representing
cells. Here and there she fitted in organs whose location she
had learned in school. Notation of tension flow revealed a ratio
of 'oral': 'anal': 'phallic' rhythms of 8:1:1. Her repertoire of
'effort' increased markedly, with lightness still prevailing. It
seemed that a new maturational spurt brought forth a control
of flow through 'effort'. But her main modes of defense, derived
from her regulation of flow by extreme stabilization, still persist as she primarily uses bound immobility, inhibition, and restriction of function.

Nancy's 'efforts' seem to operate without a foundation based
on modification of rhythms and differentiated flow regulation.
The new maturational spurt may enable Nancy to make up for
her lag in ego development. Unless this happens she may continue to use 'effort' with few variations of rhythm and in isolation from affective and mental representations.

Nancy's newfound ability to use 'effort' confirms the opinion
of observers of movement that 'efforts' have a high degree of
autonomy and may even replace flow and occur, so to speak, on
their own *(1, 34, 35, 36)*. Where 'efforts' act as physical equipment rather than as psychomotor manifestations of affective attitudes, they are almost isolated apparatus of primary autonomy that create the automated ego of a robot, without style
and ideational content.[8]

We shall know more about how 'efforts' are used in building

[8] Alexander Calder, in his machine sculpture entitled Frame, has re-created all
six elements of 'effort' of which humans are capable. He did not succeed in
combining them into one action, nor did he convey the individuality of human
action.

personality and adaptation to the wider world as the three children of my study become independent from family and school. At the age of eleven all three children still evidence a preference for rhythms of tension flow that they have favored since birth (Illustration 3), and they are still turning to methods of flow regulation adopted in early infancy. Glenda still enjoys steep rises of free flow that she uses gracefully for well-timed acceleration (Illustration 3, I). Charlie, whose combinations of rhythm and 'effort' are unusually varied and rich, still functions best from a high level of tension flow which he builds up gradually (Illustration 3, II). He still uses dazed immobility to shut out stimuli. The gradual ascent of flow intensity tends to support Charlie's deceleration when he withdraws from contact and slows down physically as well as mentally. Nancy's preference for lightness still shows traces of her neonatal limpness. Her use of strength suffers from the fact that she continues to use highly bound flow defensively (Illustration 3, III). The role these preferences played in the complex development of higher modes of functioning can best be presented through the history of Glenda's motor patterns.

Glenda's mother was very sensitive to the child's needs. The young infant slept right next to her bed so that she could hear the baby stir and be ready to respond. She picked Glenda up with gradually rising tension flow and held her for frequent short periods with lightness of effort and evenness of moderately bound flow. She blanketed her tightly but soon became concerned lest she restrict motility too much and asked my help in finding a way to keep the child warm and yet not completely restrained. She did take Glenda's fingers out of her mouth but ceased interfering because it 'made the baby angry'. She worried because the baby drank very little milk at a time and had to be fed often, but she adjusted to this schedule because 'Glenda is so little'.

Glenda's preferred biphasic rhythm consisted of a phase of steep increases and decreases of free flow, followed by phases of 'rest' which an observer who saw her as a toddler aptly called 'periods of recuperation' (3, I-6). Relaxed and graceful, Glenda did not tend to sharp reversals of flow as a newborn. She used small intensities of free and bound flow in sucking for a short time and would drop off to sleep during feeding. Back in her crib she would periodically perform like an acrobat, using sudden increases of free flow to propel herself in a supine position to the head of the crib.

Glenda's mother could develop enough steepness in ascent of flow to cope with the baby's motor feat, which she greatly admired. She attuned to the child's preferred rhythms but her own preferences for gradual ascent and steadiness of flow levels did have an influence upon the child. By the time solids were introduced, Glenda had begun to suck for longer periods of time. She was then fascinated by colorful objects at which she would stare in complete immobility. Glenda's mother respected this need, even though at times it interfered with spoon feeding. Her adjustment to the child's rhythms was most noticeable in the manner in which she presented spoonfuls of food. Each spoonful reached Glenda's mouth at the precise moment when her mouth opened to receive it. Her mother achieved this by proper timing of accelerations and was satisfied that her baby ate so quickly.

As soon as Glenda's appetite was satisfied she demanded to be put in a position in which she could stare at a red tablecloth. The mother held her on one knee to bring the child closer to the table. Using lightness and evenness of bound flow in her left arm she would at the same time change efforts and tension flow in the rest of her body to accommodate to her own needs and to those of her visitors. The staring was Glenda's own affair. Mother only provided the tablecloth and a stabilizing support. When a visiting toddler covered the tablecloth and disturbed the baby, mother reacted with gradually ascending flow intensity. Once she reached a high enough degree of intensity, she acted to restore the visual stimulus to Glenda. Perhaps she was a little late, but she taught Glenda a method of flow rise in reaction to frustration that was almost alien to the baby's repertoire of flow attributes.

Glenda's mother helped her to localize 'oral' rhythms in oral zones and encouraged independent functioning in keeping with the child's biphasic sequences. In contrast, she was neither timely nor sensitive when she localized 'anal' rhythms in the anal zone. She would become excited in what seems to me, retrospectively, a form of 'anal-sadistic' rhythm (Illustration 1, II-b) when she diapered the baby. She held up the legs in a tense, even grip. She talked in a scolding voice and then playfully spanked the baby's bottom. There was more face-to-face contact in diapering than in feeding. The mother reported with pride that Glenda soon recognized more forceful spanking as disapproval and puckered her mouth. This became a play between them rather than a clash. Although mother reported constipation in the first two or three months, she was not worried about it. Only much later, when Glenda tried to fit sitting on the pottie and getting off it into her preferred rhythm, did her mother demand that she sit there until defecation was accomplished.

The early record does not include sufficient data on rhythms other than Glenda's preferred ones, nor does it include enough clinical observations to appraise the precursors of the anal stage in Glenda's early interaction with her mother. It is apparent, however, that the maturation of visual-motor apparatus alongside the mother's tendency to use gradual ascent and even levels of bound flow and her early erotization of the anal zone, contributed to the modification of Glenda's preferred rhythmic pattern. Toward the end of the first year, when oral and anal needs normally overlap, Glenda began to rub her mother's, and later her own, underwear while engaged in autoerotic sucking (51). I once observed that the rubbing followed immediately after she touched her anus. It occurred to me then that the mother had prepared Glenda for an oro-anal centralization as a method for both gratification and tension reduction.

This method of regulation was successful in decreasing Glenda's need for biphasic functioning and was a source of comfort when her flow fluctuations became numerous at the age of four. She was then flooded by 'oral-sadistic' rhythms which were only rarely interrupted by her originally preferred 'phallic' spurts. For a time, the oral-sadistic invasion seemed to disrupt Glenda's biphasic rhythmicity. She again lost her ability or need to recuperate in frequent rest when 'phallic' thrusts in an inexhaustible succession pervaded her movements at the peak of her phallic phase. At that time, modification of her original 'phallic' rhythm brought forth sharp reversals, borrowed perhaps from the subdued 'oral-sadistic' rhythms (Illustration 3, I-b). I thought then that her phallic sadism derived its aggressive component from latent oral-sadistic wishes.

Glenda's greatest difficulty at that time was indistinct speech. She was an early talker but was unable to adjust the rise and fall of flow intensity to the length of words. She would omit word endings at points when, in her own rhythm, flow intensity dropped suddenly. In trying to regulate her speech she would use evenness of flow intensity, which promoted slurring of words into each other. Sounds would burst out as if from nowhere, when sudden ascents of free flow to high intensities broke her ability to maintain evenness of flow.

On entering school Glenda still spoke indistinctly. She was looking forward to school to the extent that she gave up sucking and rubbing of silk when told by her mother that school children did not do this. At the same time her own wish to succeed, as well as pressure from her mother and teacher, led her to subdue spurts of excitement and to transform her 'rest periods' into 'work periods'.

Throughout latency one could notice a considerable discrepancy between her motor performance in play and her deficiency in motor skills needed for school work. By the time she was ten she used all 'effort' elements in play and had acquired considerable facility in combining two and sometimes even three elements in one action. As could be predicted, her accelerations evolved easily from steep ascents of free flow, and she was equally capable of strength and lightness. She had learned to decelerate from her mother and would use this where needed. It was especially noticeable that she could move in space both directly and indirectly, but would use only precursors of these 'efforts' during work.

In writing, for instance, she had little appreciation of the space above the paper when she changed from one line to another. She would make the necessary flow changes to accomplish it but her deliberate planning caused her to decelerate. In order to write or to draw in straight lines she would use even levels of bound flow instead of the 'effort' of directness. She would erase a great deal and start anew. When she would at times become direct, a burst of free flow would soon cause her to overshoot, derail her direction, and disorganize her. She frequently regained equilibrium by an unwarranted acceleration. The first thing that seemed to come to her mind when she was confused was to 'hurry up'.

Glenda's lack of directness during work resulted from her defensive use of even bound flow, selected in emulation of her mother's preferred method of flow regulation. Her use of controlled flow changes instead of an indirect approach may have been initiated when, as a toddler, she followed her mother around the house and mirrored her movements. Her mother would wander around the house, adjusting the gas range, picking up dishes, answering the telephone, all the while turning to Glenda to praise her or to hand her a doll. All these actions required successive readjustments of flow intensity but were accomplished in a manner that conveyed wandering of attention rather than an indirect approach to objects in space.

Glenda's mother seemed to prefer lightness and deceleration. She used little strength unless challenged by a matter of great importance; she would then put her whole body into the service of strength and would frighten people into submission. In excitement she used frequent sharp reversals between free and bound flow, steep ascents and high intensity of flow. Acceleration and indirectness were less conspicuous. In a friendly mood she would approach people directly with lightness and deceleration which gave the effect of gliding. To express hostility, she would exchange lightness for strength and press her point until one had to give in.

At eleven and a half, Glenda developed a greater facility in using all 'effort' elements in a number of combinations. A maturational spurt brought about a new ability in directness and indirectness of approach, even during work periods. As a result she has become more proficient in school and the contrast between her attitude in work and in play is much less marked. She has retained her preference for acceleration and either lightness or strength. Flow notation reveals the persistence of 'phallic' rhythms, but they are far outweighed by a recent influx of 'oral' patterns. The sharp reversals from free to bound flow that characterized her 'rest' periods and work periods throughout latency have given way to smooth transitions. She seems more poised and biphasic functioning is fading. She tries to act like a young lady now and shows no evidence of the impatient and demanding behavior of her earlier years. Because of the abundance of soft transition from free to bound flow, she appears more feminine than before, but in her carriage, her choice of clothes, and her drawings she betrays her strongly phallic orientation. Her preference for steep increase of flow intensity is still in evidence, but is made less conspicuous by its incorporation into combinations of various rhythms of flow and 'effort' elements. She now uses full 'efforts' preferably in combinations that effect dabbing, flicking, and punching movements. All these contain accelerations that are initiated by sudden rises of free flow. In motor patterns and other characteristics of behavior, she shows signs of growing independence of her mother. It is too early to establish her permanent 'effort profile', too early to say wherein will lie her aptitude (*36*). We may get a better insight into the role her movement patterns played in the development of her character when we learn more about the way she uses her efforts in her relations to people.

We have seen how a mother's preference for certain qualities of tension flow and for certain 'efforts' interact with a child's congenital preferences. We have observed that maturation of apparatus makes the child partially independent of the mother. We have begun to study the role of 'effort' in the development of autonomy. We have gained some insight into the role movement patterns play in ego development. We will learn about their role in the development of object relationships when we study rhythms of 'shape' flow that underlie withdrawal and approach behavior and methods of shaping the body through which we convey our 'efforts' to others (*31*).

CONCLUSION

The rhythms of the neonate's movement contain the *Anlage* for expression of drive and affect and for their regulation as well.

Analysis of rhythms of flow of tension reveals an alternation between two basic elements, free flow and bound flow. This alternation reflects the changing balance between agonistic and antagonistic muscle groups. Imbalance of these muscle groups results in movement that brings the individual into contact with the outer world; their balance causes immobility which withdraws the individual from contact. Extreme imbalance exposes him to the dangers of a clash between himself and the outer world, but extreme balance exposes him to dangers from within. Immobility, apathy, or rigidity prevent us from using the resources of our body for survival.

The polarity of free and bound flow is a quality of organic life from which Freud derived his concepts of polarities of pleasure and unpleasure, of life and death instincts (8). It reflects two trends in regulation. One is a basic trend toward the world around us that prompts us to use the resources of nature for our survival. The other, antithetical trend protects us from the dangers of too great an exposure to reality.

But rhythms of tension flow contain a more complex regulatory mechanism in the qualities of free and bound flow that are also capable of change. Flow of tension varies as its intensity increases or decreases, remains steady or fluctuates, and changes gradually or suddenly. These polarities of flow attributes form the basis for all the varieties of movement possible to us in our accommodation to the environment and our defenses against it.

All possible rhythms of tension flow seem to be available to the neonate. But he hardly has any ability to organize them for adaptation or defense. To do this he needs the combined influence of reality (and its foremost exponent—his mother) and the maturation of his organ systems. We too easily forget that apparatus and structures, be they somatic or psychic, are regulatory systems (5, 18, 40), and we burden ourselves too much by trying to establish when psychic functioning begins. It seems that all functions become mobilized at birth when the neonate becomes exposed to external stimuli and begins to function autonomously.

In the basic rhythms of alternations between free and bound flow, we recognize a regulation familiar to us from primary process functioning. The primitive archaic regulations of the id shift from displacement to condensation of psychic energy. When the ego gains access to the regulation of frequencies of their repetition, in various degrees of intensities and at various rates of increase, condensation and displacement become subject to the laws of secondary process functioning (27).

Frequency of repetition, degree of intensity, and rate of increase of flow, free and bound, combine to form rhythms that are appropriate for need satisfaction in particular zones of the body. In this process we see a model for the operation of drives which are the psychic representatives of needs. The regulation of quality and quantity of free and bound discharge in the id is dependent on rhythmic changes in various organs of the body. Individual differences are expressed in the frequency and combination of these 'organ' rhythms. These individual differences contribute to the individuality in the central organization of rhythm in the nervous system. They appear to be the core of the id-ego organization from which individual traits of the ego emerge (12, 18).

Analysis of rhythms of tension flow suggests that rhythmic discharge is characteristic of the id. The id becomes a mere 'seething cauldron' when rhythm ceases and boundness prevents discharge (16, 19); conversely, it becomes an 'erupting volcano' when rhythm ceases and free discharge becomes boundless. These are primitive regulatory mechanisms that are used throughout life as emergency measures. Analysis of attributes of tension flow suggests that the regulation of frequency, intensity, and rate of discharge, which are originally determined by the confluence of rhythms of different organ systems, is taken over by the ego. The ego not only 'transforms the id's will into actions . . .' but also mediates between the organism and its milieu. Organ systems that are specifically designed to receive stimuli from outside the body oppose rhythmic discharge and promote flow stabilization and delay in repetition. The body ego evolves from the id as it incorporates the noncognitive kinesthetic perception of tension rhythms. To the degree that it incorporates acoustic and visual perceptions the ego becomes the exponent of continuity of environmental forces.

Maturation of psychomotor apparatus that serves adjustment to the environment supports and further differentiates ego functioning. Motor patterns, which are designed to cope with forces of our environment, are 'efforts' that we use in our adjustment to space, gravity, and time. The complex functions of the ego include several modes of motor discharge that develop in successive stages: rhythms of tension flow appropriate to specific tasks are localized in specific functional zones; elements and attributes of tension flow are selected in the service of actions that require delay in repetition; fine gradation of flow attributes adds melody to rhythmic movements; rhythms become subordinated to adaptive aims in 'efforts'.

Differentiation of drives is contingent on differentiation of rhythms to conform to optimal modes of discharge in zones in which specific concrete transactions occur between the body and its milieu. When drive discharge is thus localized and its rhythm becomes truly functional, there begins a specific ego-controlled drive organization. This becomes possible only when the mother lends to the child her own methods of regulation and mediates between him and reality before a constant ego takes over this function and makes the child independent. During these transactions the child's original endowment becomes modified; within the complex modified functioning of the adult we may, however, detect traces of inborn traits that we have observed in the newborn.

GLOSSARY

Attributes of free and bound flow are qualities of flow that depend on the fre
quency of changes, the degree of their intensity, and the rate of increase o
decrease. The intensity of tension may fluctuate or remain even for a time, i
may decrease or increase, it may rise or abate gradually or steeply.

Centralization: A method of flow regulation in which all parts of the body
simultaneously or successively, undergo flow changes in consonance with a
localized functional activity. For instance, the whole body of a drummer con
tributes to the actions of the arms.

Effort: A motion factor that expresses the changes in our attitudes toward space
gravity, and time.

Effort elements are direct or indirect in relation to space, strong or light in rela
tion to weight, increasing or decreasing speed in relation to time.

Elements of flow are free, uninhibited flow in movement that cannot be easily
stopped at will; and bound, inhibited flow that can be easily stopped at any
point of movement.

Flow of tension: A motion factor that pertains to the sequence of fluency and
restraint in the state of muscles in movement and rest. Laban refers to it a
'flow of effort' because efforts arise from flow and use it for their adaptive aims

Flow regulation organizes flow changes in the service of functions.

Localization is a mechanism of flow regulation which initiates and maintains zone
specific patterns of flow changes in functionally related parts of the body s
that a sucking rhythm becomes dominant in the mouth region or a rhythm
appropriate to grasping in the hand.

Melody of movement results from a flow regulation in which flow intensity i
graduated in a selected sequence.

Modification of rhythms of flow occurs when several rhythms combine with each
other, or when one or more flow qualities of a rhythmic pattern are change
through flow regulation. A child may decrease the rate of rise of tension in
sucking because of a confluence of 'oral' and 'anal' rhythms, or he may do s
to conform to the rhythm with which milk is released from the nipple.

Modulation of flow: A regulation by fine graduation of intensities.

Phrasing of rhythmic patterns: Organization of sequences of selected rhythms o
tension flow and effort, in a manner characteristic for an individual.

Redistribution of flow: A flow regulation through which flow elements are
changed in various parts of the body to initiate, maintain, change, or stop a
functional activity.

Rhythm: Periodic repetition of variations in one or more quality. In regula
rhythms, the intervals between variations and the modes of variations are con
sistently the same.

Rhythm of tension flow: Periodic alternation between free and bound flow i
simple rhythmic patterns to which is added a variation of flow attributes in
complex rhythms. Regular stimuli evoke pure rhythms in which intervals be
tween variation and the degree of change in frequency, quantity, and rate o
increase or decrease of free and bound flow are consistent.

Selection of flow elements and their attributes: Flow regulation by planned selection of flow qualities in adaptation to reality; for instance, choosing even bound flow to reach a small object. This type of flow regulation is a part-function of effort and its precursor.

Stabilization: Flow regulation that decreases the frequency of flow fluctuations. Complete stabilization leads to immobility in all parts of the body. Partial stabilization reduces flow changes in certain parts of the body to prevent interference with localized motor discharge.

Subordination of flow to efforts: Flow regulation in various parts of the body by which sequences of flow changes are adapted to the effort elements chosen.

REFERENCES

1. BARTENIEFF, IRMA: *Effort Observation and Effort Assessment in Rehabilitation.* (Lecture at the National Notation Conference.) New York: Dance Notation Bureau, 1962.

2. BONAPARTE, MARIE: *Time and the Unconscious.* Int. J. Psa., XXI, 1940, pp. 427-468.

3. CALL, JUSTIN D.: *Newborn Approach Behavior and Early Ego Development.* Int. J. Psa., XLV, 1964, pp. 286-295.

4. DEUTSCH, FELIX, Editor: *On the Mysterious Leap from the Mind to the Body. A Workshop Study on the Theory of Conversion.* New York: International Universities Press, Inc., 1959.

5. ESCALONA, SIBYLLE: *The Impact of Psychoanalysis Upon Child Psychology.* J. Nervous & Mental Disease, CXXVI, 1958.

6. FREUD, ANNA: *The Ego and the Mechanisms of Defense* (1936). New York: International Universities Press, Inc., 1946.

7. FREUD: *Three Essays on the Theory of Sexuality* (1901-1905). Standard Edition, VII.

8. ———: *Beyond the Pleasure Principle* (1920). Standard Edition, XVIII.

9. ———: *The Ego and the Id* (1923) Standard Edition, XIX.

10. ———: *A Note Upon the Mystic Writing Pad* (1924). Standard Edition, XIX.

11. ———: *The Economic Problem of Masochism* (1924). Standard Edition, XIX.

12. ———: *Analysis Terminable and Interminable* (1937). Standard Edition, XXIII.

13. ——— and BREUER, JOSEF: *Studies on Hysteria* (1893-1895). Standard Edition, II.

14. FRIES, MARGARET: *Factors in Character Development.* Amer. J. Orthopsychiatry, VII, 1937, pp. 142-181.

15. ———: Some Hypotheses on the Role of the Congenital Activity Type in Personality and Development. In: *The Psychoanalytic Study of the Child, Vol. XIII.* New York: International Universities Press, Inc., 1958, pp.48-64.

16. GILL, MERTON M.: On Topography and Structure in Psychoanalysis. In: *Psychological Issues, V.* New York: International Universities Press, Inc., 1963.

17. GREENACRE, PHYLLIS: Problems of Infantile Neurosis. In: *The Psychoanalytic Study of the Child, Vol. IX*. New York: International Universities Press, Inc., 1954, pp. 18-24.

18. HARTMANN, HEINZ: *Ego Psychology and the Problem of Adaptation*. New York: International Universities Press, Inc., 1958.

19. ———: The Mutual Influences in the Development of Ego and Id. In: *Essays on Ego Psychology*. New York: International Universities Press, Inc., 1964.

20. HOFFER, WILLI: Mouth, Hand and Ego Integration. In: *The Psychoanalytic Study of the Child, Vols. III/IV*. New York: International Universities Press, Inc., 1949, pp. 18-23.

21. ———: Development of the Body Ego. In: *The Psychoanalytic Study of the Child, Vol. V*. New York: International Universities Press, Inc., 1950, pp. 49-56.

22. HOLLOS, STEFAN: *Über das Zeitgefühl*. Int. Ztschr. f. Psa., VIII, 1922, pp. 421-439.

23. JACOBSON, EDITH: The Affects and Their Pleasure-Unpleasure Qualities in Relation to the Psychic Discharge Processes. In: *Drives, Affects, Behavior*. Edited by Rudolph M. Loewenstein. New York: International Universities Press, Inc., 1953.

24. KAPLAN, ELISABETH B.: *Reflections Regarding Psychomotor Activities During the Latency Period*. Panel on Latency. Meeting of the American Psychoanalytic Association, 1964.

25. (KESTENBERG) SILBERPFENNIG, J.: *Contribution to the Problems of Eye Movements. 1. Eye Movements in Insulin-Coma*. Confinia Neurologica, I, 1938, pp. 188-200.

26. KESTENBERG, JUDITH S.: *Early Reactions to Tensions*. Read at Meeting of the New York Psychoanalytic Society, 1945.

27. ———: *Note on Ego Development*. Int. J. Psa., XXXIV, 1953, pp. 1-12.

28. ———: *History of an 'Autistic' Child*. J. Child Psychiatry, II, 1935, pp. 5-52.

29. ———: Problems of Infantile Neurosis. In: *The Psychoanalytic Study of the Child, Vol. IX*. New York: International Universities Press, Inc., 1954, pp. 18-24.

30. ———: *The Role of Movement Patterns in Development. I. Rhythms of Movement*. This QUARTERLY, XXXIV, 1965, pp. 1-36.

31. ———: *The Role of Movement Patterns in Development. III. Shape, Flow, Shaping*. In preparation.

32. KHAN, M. MASUD R.: *Ego Distortion, Cumulative Trauma, and the Role of Reconstruction*. Int. J. Psa., XLV, 1964, pp. 272-279.

33. KRIS, ERNST: Some Comments and Observations on Early Auto-erotic Activities. In: *The Psychoanalytic Study of the Child, Vol. V*. New York: International Universities Press, Inc., 1961, pp. 95-116.

34. LABAN, RUDOLF: *The Mastery of Movement*. Second edition. Revised by L. Ullman. London: MacDonald & Evans, Ltd., 1960.

35. ——— and LAWRENCE, F.: *Effort*. London: MacDonald & Evans, Ltd., 1947.

36. LAMB, WARREN: *Aptitude for Management: Its Relation to Executive Health*. The Manager, J. British Inst. of Management, XXVII/2. London: Management Publications Ltd., 1959, pp. 102-103.

37. MOSONYI, DESIDERIUS: *Die irrationalen Grundlagen der Musik*. Imago, XXI, 1935, pp. 207-226.

38. PIAGET, JEAN: *The Child's Conception of Physical Causality*. New York: Harcourt Brace & Co., 1930.

39. PRATT, KARL C.: The Neonate. In: *Manual of Child Psychology*. Edited by L. Carmichael. New York: John Wiley & Sons, Inc., 1946.

40. RAPAPORT, DAVID: *On the Psychoanalytic Theory of Thinking*. Int. J. Psa., XXXI, 1950.

41. ——— and GILL, MERTON M.: *The Points of View and Assumptions of Metapsychology*. Int. J. Psa., XL, 1959.

42. RUCKMICK, C. A.: *The Rhythmical Experience from the Systematic Point of View*. Amer. J. Psychology, XXXIX, 1923.

43. RUSSEL, JOAN: *Modern Dance in Education*. London: MacDonald & Evans, Ltd., 1958.

44. SCHILDER, PAUL: *The Image and Appearance of the Human Body*. Psyche Monographs No. 4. London: Kegal Paul, Trench, Trubner & Co., 1935.

45. SPIELREIN, SABINE: *Die Zeit im unterschwelligen Seelenleben*. Imago, IX, 1923, pp. 300-317.

46. SPITZ, RENÉ A.: *Wiederholung, Rhythmus und Langeweile*. Imago, XXIII, 1937, pp. 171-196.

47. STAERKE, AUGUST: *Entwicklungs Phasen der psychischen Motilität*. Beiheft der Int. Ztschr. f. Psa., IV, 1918.

48. ———: *Über Tanzen, Schlagen, Küssen usw*. Imago, XII, 1926, pp. 268-272.

49. STERN, MAX: *Prototypes of Defenses*. Int. J. Psa., XLV, 1964, pp. 296-297.

50. ———: *Prototypes of Mental Phenomena*. Read at Meeting of the New York Psychoanalytic Association, 1963.

51. WINNICOTT, D. W.: *Transitional Objects and Transitional Phenomena*. Int. J. Psa., XXXIV, 1953.

52. WOLFF, P.: *Observations of Newborn Infants*. Psychosomatic Med., XXI, 1959, pp. 110-118.

THE ROLE OF MOVEMENT PATTERNS IN DEVELOPMENT

III. THE CONTROL OF SHAPE

BY JUDITH S. KESTENBERG, M.D. (NEW YORK)

To serve as the prototype for all others, there is one basic developmental line which has received attention from analysts from the beginning. This is the sequence which leads from the newborn's utter dependence on maternal care to the young adult's emotional and material self-reliance—a sequence for which the successive stages of libido development (oral, anal, phallic) merely form the inborn maturational base. . . . When the child's muscular actions come under the control of the sensible ego instead of serving the impulses in the id, this is another important step towards socialization.

—ANNA FREUD *(18)*

Muscular actions are the instruments that change the relation between the self[1] and the world of objects. Complex as are these relations in civilized adults, they have a basic rhythmical structure that is found in plants, animals, and human infants. Laban's poetic description captures the quality of this rhythm: 'Each movement is conceived and born, grows and shrinks,

From the Department of Psychiatry, Division of Psychoanalytic Education, State University of New York, Downstate Medical Center, Brooklyn, New York, and from the Long Island Jewish Hospital, New Hyde Park, New York.

A number of ideas about shape crystallized in discussions with the members of the Movement Study Group (Dr. Jay Berlowe, Arnhild Buehlte, Godfrey Cobliner, Ph.D., Dr. Hershey Marcus, Forrestine Paulay, and Dr. Esther Robbins). The continuous guidance of Warren Lamb and helpful discussions with Irma Bartenieff of New York, and Lillian Harmel, Marion North, and Valerie Preston of England are gratefully acknowledged.

[1] Throughout this paper the term 'self' refers to the subject as distinguished from the object.

and finally fades into the past and nothingness' *(35)*. As the amœba extends its pseudopodia, it grows in space and thus comes closer to the source of nutriment in the environment; when it shrinks it increases the distance between its body and the objects in space and in a sense comes closer to itself *(19)*. The body of the amœba changes its shape in a rhythmic sequence of growing and shrinking in which the protoplasm flows outward and inward. This 'flow of shape' is the apparatus of approach and withdrawal. The changing conformations of the body evoke responsive feeling tones as the flow of shape interacts with the changing states of tension (the 'flow of tension' [*30*]) in the organism.

Rhythms of tension-flow are sequences of fluency and restraint in the state of the muscles in various parts of the body. They are apparatus for discharge of drives through motor channels. Rhythms of shape-flow organize the relationship of body parts in such a way that drives can be satisfied in transactions with objects. In successive developmental phases regulations of tension-flow and shape-flow come under the control of the ego. Regulation of tension-flow aids drive differentiation; regulation of shape-flow contributes to the differentiation of self and objects. In later development, ego attitudes to space, gravity, and time, expressed through 'efforts', control the flow of tension. At the same time, shape-flow becomes subordinated to selective shaping of movement in the dimensions and planes in which transactions with objects take place.

In this paper I will attempt to correlate the development of movement patterns that serve affective object relations with psychoanalytic theories of the genesis of object relations.

Freud *(20)* in his early formulation of the nature of drives, distinguishes between the source of a drive, its force, its aim, and the object by which the aim can be fulfilled. Bodily needs that give impetus to the drive also determine its aim. The object, whether it is the body itself or something outside it, is at first found in what seems a haphazard way. We have been at a loss to define the nature of self and objects during the phase of primary masochism (primary narcissism) and primary identification *(26)*. During the transition from objectless autism to the self-centered relation with the anaclitic object, the emergent body boundaries are blurred and the rudimentary body image merges with a near object *(5, 26, 39, 40, 47)*. This merging becomes disrupted by repeated experiences of separation from the object. From then on there is continuous yearning for closeness to the object and throughout life the periphery of the body retains a double representation,—self and need-satisfying object. The center of the body remains the core of self-representation, but its periphery continues to be the no-man's land in which self and object are doubly represented. The 'near space', that area just surrounding the periphery, belongs to the body image as well as to the outside space through which the hand passes to reach other parts of the body *(47)*. In this very near space, closeness to intimate objects reaches its climax in brief experiences of fusion characteristic of early relationships.

Because of the intermittent nature of anaclitic relationships *(17)*, availability of the object is essential for drive satisfaction. The basic characteristic of the object at that time is that it appears when needed, that it is within reach. As the child begins to understand the distance between self and object, the 'near space' can be distinguished from another space that also belongs to the self—'reach space'.[2] Once the object of the drive becomes constant *(17, 18, 23)*, the child selectively directs movement toward the object. As he gains control over the locomotor apparatus, he can move his whole body in search of the object in the general space.

Recalling the visual image of the object substitutes for immediate reaching or moving in the general space. The image is often projected into space at the border between reach space and general space; this gives the illusion that the object is

---

[2] Laban *(35)* called this the 'kinesphere', the personal space that 'remains constant in relation to the body when we move away from the original stance; it travels with the body in the general space'.

within reach. However, the image of the absent object cannot forever substitute for the real object. The seeking of the loved one in farther and farther domains of the wider space comes to a peak in adolescence in the almost mystic oceanic feeling of reaching out to the universe and growing out into the horizon.

The rhythm of 'shrinking and growing' provides the motor apparatus for the continuous rhythmic transformation of narcissistic libido into object libido and vice versa (*19, 21, 22, 26, 38, 50*). The rhythmic flow of shape constitutes the framework for the flowing of libido and aggression between self and object. As development progresses, self and object representations are guided by the reciprocal relation of body shape to the shape of the space around it. When we feel larger, the world narrows; when we feel taller it seems smaller; and when we protrude into it, it appears hollow. These shapes of feelings (*27, 46*) differentiate into affective images of self and object at the same time as directions, dimensions, and configurations in space come to serve transactions between self and objects. Growing and shrinking of body shapes can be observed in all forms of approach and withdrawal, such as turning to objects and away from them, 'standing up' to them or 'bowing down', following or retreating, seeking or fleeing.

Hermann (*24*) drew upon observations of primates and analyses of adults to postulate special drives of clinging and seeking. Balint (*2, 3*) expanded this classification into phases and types of 'ocnophilic' clinging and 'philobatic' seeking of friendly expanses. Both authors recognized that they were dealing with an organizing principle that pervades behavior throughout phylogeny and ontogeny. Clinging and seeking are subphases of the ubiquitous rhythm of shape-flow which results from the alternation of two opposing tendencies of the organism: flexion, which brings body parts closer to each other and maintains the organism in 'near space', and extension, which separates joints from each other and moves the organism into 'reach space'. Automatisms of seeking, observable in young animals and human neonates, are part of the neurophysiological apparatus for positioning body parts in relation to each other and for orientation to objects *(4, 10, 42, 43, 51)*. Spontaneous and reflexive rooting alternates direction before contact with the nipple is established *(30, 51)*. After satiation the infant draws away from the mother's body; pushing out the nipple and turning away from the breast terminates contact. All these centrifugal and centripetal movements change the shape of the body which seems to grow toward the outside and to shrink inward.

Schneirla *(48)* used the example of the local flow of the amœba's protoplasm toward weak light and away from strong noxious stimuli to show that the adaptive responses of approach and withdrawal contribute to the survival of the species. Although he looked upon approach and withdrawal as apparatus for interaction with the environment, he also applied these terms to motivated behavior that includes ego functions. The rhythm of growing and shrinking of body shape is contained in approach and withdrawal behavior in all levels of development. It occurs in response to salutary or noxious, external or internal, stimuli in relation to external objects and in relation to the infant's own body. Growing is related to intake and shrinking to expulsion, as exemplified in the rhythms of heartbeat, breathing, feeding, and elimination. The outward direction of growing and inward direction of shrinking conform to the fact that life depends on the beneficial sources of the environment and avoidance of death depends on the organism's capacity to shrink and avoid or expel the noxious *(22, 26)*.

In his extensive research, Schneirla *(48)* found that the young mammal's 'approach behavior' is correlated with vegetative changes characterized by smoothly running continuous processes. Conversely 'withdrawal behavior' is correlated with changes in the sympathetic nervous system, characterized by interruptive processes. In observation of movement patterns one finds an affinity between 'growing' of body shape and free flow of tension (smoothly running continuous processes), and an affinity between 'shrinking' of body shape and bound flow of tension (interruptive processes).[8] These observations also suggest that growing of body shape combined with free flow of tension is conducive to the outward discharge of libido; shrinking of body shape combined with bound flow seems best suited for the discharge of aggression inward (22). But even in the newborn, the rhythms of shape-flow and tension-flow combine in a more complex way that does not necessarily follow the principle of affinity between 'growing' and free flow or 'shrinking' and bound flow. Under conditions of optimal maternal care, the regulation of tension-flow and shape-flow is gradually taken over by the ego, which maintains an equilibrium between the discharge of quantities of libido and aggression zonally,[4] inward and outward, to the self and objects.

HIERARCHY OF MOVEMENT PATTERNS

Rhythms of tension-flow and shape-flow can be noted in all movement. Regulations of tension-flow and shape-flow organize these discharge forms in the service of functions.

The rhythm of tension-flow consists of alternations between free and bound movements (30). The rhythm of shape-flow consists of alternations between growing and shrinking of body shape (36). The term 'shape' pertains to the appearance of the body and its parts in extension and flexion and is not to be confused with actual changes in size or postures (see footnote 5 below). Both tension-flow and shape-flow depend on the in-

[8] The correlation of 'approach' with low intensity stimuli and 'withdrawal' with high intensity stimuli, which Schneirla postulates, parallels Sherrington's (49) principle of differential and antagonistic systems in skeletal muscle function. This principle links extensor dominance with weak stimulation and flexor dominance with strong stimulation. Our data show that 'growing' is based on extensor dominance and 'shrinking' on flexor dominance.

[4] The term 'zonal discharge' pertains to forms of discharge appropriate to the functions of the anatomical zone in which the discharge takes place. For example, rhythms of sucking, chewing, biting, and speaking are forms of discharge in the oral zone. When an inappropriate discharge form invades a zone— for instance, when an 'anal' rhythm is used for activities in the oral zone—it interferes with optimal functioning (29, 30).

terplay between agonistic and antagonistic sets of muscles and on gamma-regulation in individual muscles, governed by the reticular system *(4)*. These apparatus serve drive discharge in such a way that the rhythm of tension-flow conforms to specific zonal needs while the rhythm of shape-flow directs the discharge outward and inward. Tension-flow is a carrier for the flow of pleasure and unpleasure; shape-flow gives structure to these feelings so that we can recognize them as specific moods (feeling expansive or constricted, big or small, full or empty).

Intrinsic in the neonate's rhythms are regulatory mechanisms which gradually come under the control of the ego. Regulation of tension-flow pertains to control over sequences of free and bound flow, over frequency of fluctuation in intensity of tension, and over the degree and rate of its increase and decrease (intensity factors of tension-flow). Regulation of shape-flow pertains to the control over sequences of centrifugal and centripetal movements which make the shape of the body appear larger or smaller. A more advanced regulation of shape-flow consists in controlled selection of the horizontal, vertical, and sagittal dimensions of the body in which shape widens or narrows, lengthens or shortens, bulges or hollows (dimensional factors of shape-flow). At the same time as the shape of the body changes during movement, the whole body or its parts traverses space in lines or loops, in large or small degrees, with sharp reversals or smooth curves (design factors of shape-flow). Regulation of design factors permits a limited selection of ways by which body shape changes through movement. All these regulations underlie the mechanisms through which the ego distributes quantities of libido and aggression and maintains an affective equilibrium between self and objects *(7)*.

Successive adaptations to space, gravity, and time lead to controlled selections of qualities of tension-flow best suited to reach objects in space, to handle them according to their weight, and to get to them on time. These are precursors of adaptation through 'effort' *(30)*. Gradually movement becomes subservient to concepts of 'where, what, and when' *(35)* as mature patterns of 'effort', governed by the reality principle, subordinate rhythms of tension-flow to adaptive aims of the ego. A prototype of an aggressive action is punching, in which direct, strong, and fast 'effort' elements use appropriate rhythms of tension-flow to produce the desired effect. For example, a pure or modified 'phallic' rhythm could be used for punching but an 'oral' type of rhythm would not be suitable. A prototype of an indulging action is floating, in which indirect, light, and slow 'effort' elements control the flow of tension to make it compatible with aim-inhibited discharge of libido *(30, 35, 36)*.

Successive adjustment to objects leads to controlled selections of spatial directions and movement in spatial planes. The child begins to shape his body to conform to such prescriptions of direction as 'to the side and across to the other side' which evolves from 'widening and narrowing'; 'up and down' which evolves from 'lengthening and shortening'; and 'forward and backward' which evolves from 'bulging and hollowing'. The highest form of regulation of shape-flow is achieved through active 'shaping' of the space between self and objects; variations in body shapes become automatic as they are incorporated into the adaptive aim of the ego to change spatial relations.

'Directional shaping' evolves from regulation of changes in the dimensions of the body that are extended into space. When space is conceived as multidimensional, a complex relationship to objects in space is expressed through meaningful interactions in the horizontal, vertical, and sagittal planes through spreading in space or enclosing it, ascending or descending, advancing or retiring. While 'directional shaping' erects a bridge between oneself and the object, 'shaping of space in planes' creates a two or three dimensional spatial configuration which gives a complex design to the relationship. Shaping of space in planes evolves from regulations of dimensions and design used in the flow of shape and from control over spatial directions.

As is the case with 'effort' elements, in 'shaping' too there are many possible combinations. There is an affinity between certain 'effort' elements and related elements in 'shaping'—for instance, between exertion of strength and downward motions or lightness and rising. An integration of related patterns of movement reflects a balance between aims of drives and phase adequate relating to objects.

Already in infancy one can distinguish between regulations which aid localization of discharge in one part of the body and those which promote centralization of discharge in which all parts of the body, simultaneously or successively, move in consonance with each other *(30)*. These early regulations differentiate into movements, called 'gestures' and 'postures' *(36)*. The term 'gesture', as used here, is not to be confused with gesticulation or with the learned modes of substituting stylized patterns for words; it denotes movements that are confined to one part of the body (such as head, arm, leg). The term 'posture' is not to be confused with a static disposition of the body and its parts that corresponds most closely to what in this paper is referred to as 'shape'[5]; 'posture' as used here denotes a dynamic pattern of movement involving the whole body and using identical elements of 'effort' or 'shaping' throughout. In precursors of postural movement, all parts of the body move in similar rhythms of tension-flow or shape-flow. Postural move-

---

[5] Deutsch's pioneering work on 'analytic posturology' can be better correlated with the material presented in this paper if the term 'shape' is substituted for the term 'posture' *(12, 13, 14)*. Deutsch showed conclusively that preferred body shapes express modes of self-representations and that changes of direction in movement indicate changes in relation to objects.

It is important to keep to Laban's and Lamb's terminology wherever possible, as our notation and interpretation of movement profiles is based on their work. Variations of effort and shaping elements in postures and gestures are notated; 'effort' and 'shape' profiles are used in conformity with Lamb's specifications *(36)*. Conceptualizations of Laban and his pupils are also used, but our different orientation leads to a psychoanalytic interpretation of movement patterns and profiles *(32)*. The notation and interpretation of rhythms of tension-flow and shape-flow is unique to the Movement Study Group in Sands Point. Rhythms of tension-flow have been classified in previous papers *(29, 30, 31)* in accordance with optimal modes of zonal discharge.

The notation of rhythms of shape-flow was devised by Forrestine Paulay and the author. The experience with the interpretation of these rhythms is too new to warrant a comprehensive presentation of their role in forming shapes of object relationships *(27, 46)*.

ments occur in states of high motivation or total involvement with an object.

The consistent use of 'effort' and 'shaping' patterns in postures is ushered in by maturation of apparatus for total body coördination. This occurs in adolescence, at the same time as the influx of high quantities of sex specific hormones. Postural movement through effort and shaping represents the motor component of processes which lead to identity formation in adolescence. To the degree that the adult individual is able to function consistently in states of high and low motivation, he uses the same effort and shaping patterns in 'postures' as in 'gestures'. Discrepancies between patterns used in postures and gestures reveal areas of conflict and point the way to appraisal of defense mechanisms from observation of movement.

Control of the environment through 'efforts' and 'shaping' derives its affective components from regulations of tension-flow and shape-flow. Advanced regulation of tension-flow gives melody to movement and advanced regulation of shape-flow achieves a harmonious balance between shapes of various parts of the body. When tension-flow and shape-flow are controlled by integrated patterns of effort and shaping in postures and gestures, movement becomes a composition in which themes are expressed through efforts and orchestration is provided through shaping.

RHYTHMS OF SHAPE-FLOW AND TENSION-FLOW

There is a continuous interdependence between tension of the body and its shape in rest, and between rhythms of tension-flow and shape-flow in mobility. The boundaries of the infant's body are outlined by the distribution of tension in his skeletal muscles. The mobility of the neonate's shoulder and hip joints is hampered by the boundness of muscles in these areas. His arms are still close to his chest and his legs close to his abdomen. The newborn's shape appears not only narrow and hollow but also shorter than it actually is. In states of mobility, his limbs move in all directions but his proximal joints participate only to a limited degree. Consecutive changes in shape can be noted as the newborn folds and unfolds, coils and uncoils, bends and stretches in regular or irregular rhythms. His mouth and hands seem to exert a magnetic attraction toward each other, but they rarely maintain closeness. An influx of free flow, which is one element of the rhythm of tension-flow, pulls hand and mouth apart. In the lower part of the body, knees bend and stretch, coming closer to the abdomen and getting farther away from it, at more or less regular intervals. The intervals between growing and shrinking of body shape are determined by the degree to which bound and free flow can be maintained in the periphery and the center of the body. In states of excitement, centrifugal and centripetal movements increase in frequency and amplitude at the same time as free and bound flow alternate more frequently and increase in intensity. In end-phases of excitement, the frequency and amplitude of growing and shrinking decrease. Depending on the state of tension in the infant's muscles, he may lapse into rigid immobility or flaccid limpness. Rigid tension in the periphery of the body sharpens its outlines; flabbiness softens the body contours.

With the emergence of psychic awareness, both 'growing' and 'shrinking' become associated with pleasurable sensations, reflecting the excitement of mounting tension and the relief of subsiding tension. Freud (22) pointed out that the relation between intensity of excitation and pleasure-unpleasure qualities is not a simple one. He suspected that the amount of increase and diminution of excitation in a given period of time may be the decisive determinant of qualities of feelings. The intensity factors of tension-flow and the dimensional factors of shape-flow combine in various ways from which emerge various qualities of pleasure and pain as well as other associated affects.

To illustrate the relationship between tension-flow and shape-flow rhythms and ranges of feeling the infant may experience, it is useful to explore how these factors operate in the breathing of adults.

During normal breathing the attributes of tension-flow and

shape-flow change minimally. Yet we can observe that we inhale in free flow which gradually goes over into bound flow to become free again in exhalation and bound or neutral in the pause that follows it. In inhalation we widen, lengthen, and bulge; in exhalation we narrow, shorten, and become hollow. When we take a deep breath we may experience a feeling of exhilaration; exhaling after holding of breath brings on a feeling of relief. Prolonged breath-holding in inspiration goes along with exaggerated growing of body and a high degree of boundness and extensor tension. These changes can evoke sensations of bursting which merge with feelings of rage and anxiety. This type of anxiety may lead to fears of falling apart, becoming fragmented and losing body parts, and may eventually culminate in castration fear. In expiration prolonged breath holding goes along with exaggerated shrinking of body shape and a high degree of boundness and flexor tension. These may evoke sensations of being knotted up or wound up inside, as if one's own aggression turning inward were taking on a shape. In sudden expiration, an abrupt decrease of tension and flaccid shrinking can evoke feelings of deflation, collapse, and emptiness. Rhythms of shape-flow in which exaggerated shrinking recurs frequently can lead to a variety of feelings of agitated and flat depression, of fears of becoming smaller and separated from objects.

Growing and shrinking of body shape help to localize the inside and the outside of the body; at the same time, feelings of being propelled outward or pulled inward outline the directions that develop into vectors of intentional movement. The postural image of the body (47) becomes the basis for shapes of self-representation (27, 46). Tension-flow is related to basic moods of being carefree in free flow and constrained in bound flow (30); shape-flow contributes to the specificity of moods and self-representations. Feeling expansive and generous, constricted and miserly, big and elated, small and subdued, full and proud, empty and insignificant are all derived from various degrees and vectors of sensations of growing and shrinking. The end less variety of feeling tones and shades of self-esteem which arise from tension-flow and shape-flow rhythms in turn influence these rhythms.

Changes in tension-flow and shape-flow and in their attributes (intensity factor of tension, dimensional and design factors of shape) unite to produce complex patterns of movement that can be noted in the newborn, even though he has neither control over tension nor over spatial dimensions. His limbs, free or bound, traverse space in the horizontal, vertical, and sagittal dimensions and, in so doing, proceed in lines or loops and in high or low amplitudes, turning in sharp angles or soft curves. All these qualities vary not only from moment to moment but also from limb to limb. The neonate's preferences for specific combinations of tension-flow and shape-flow rhythms mark his individuality. Certain elements and attributes of tension-flow lend themselves to expression of aggression while others are more conducive to discharge of libido. Elements and attributes of shape-flow give to this discharge direction and design through which precursors of expression of affect become meaningful to the onlooker. From the individuality of these apparatus for drive discharge that can be noted in the newborn, we may be able to appraise his drive endowment and his affective potential for relating to people before psychic differentiation provides a basis for psychological assessment *(30, 32)*.

Bound flow of tension gives a 'fighting' quality to movement and free flow 'indulges' in mobility *(35)*, characteristic for discharge of libido. The affinity of bound flow and shrinking, and free flow and growing of body shape has been mentioned before. There is also an affinity between attributes of tension-flow and shape-flow: 1. Maintenance of even levels of tension combines easily with narrowing linear movements, high intensity with shortening of shape and high amplitudes, sudden rises of tension with hollowing and sharpness of angles. (These combinations are characteristic for discharge of aggression inward.) 2. Fluctuations of intensity of tension combine often with widening sinuous movements, low intensity of tension with lengthening of body shape and low amplitudes, gradual rise of tension with bulging and curving movements. (These combinations are characteristic for discharge of libido outward.) It is self-evident that all these factors unite in numerous ways and there is no strict adherence to rules of affinity. However, movement regulated by the principle of affinity between motion factors is clearer and easier to describe and easier to correlate with moods and feeling tones through which we recognize the operation of aggressive or libidinal drives in relation to objects. The following correlations of coördinated attributes of tension-flow and shape-flow with corresponding moods will serve as a rough classification of affecto-motor qualities of object relations. In each example an attempt is made to show how feelings related to a set of motion factors can alter when free flow changes into bound flow, and vice versa. Refinement of feeling tones contributed by the affinity of design factors is also mentioned.

1. Even intensity of tension, combined with narrowing of shape, may provide an atmosphere of steady enclosing in free flow and constrictive holding in bound flow. Where the narrowing divides space in a straight line, it adds the feeling tone of restrictive finality.

2. Fluctuating intensity of tension, combined with widening of shape, promises a wide scope in exploring and considering the needs of others. But when too many fluctuations of free flow predominate one may get the impression of erratic meandering or when bound flow is dominant of uneasy squirming. Loops or twists can add the tone of playfulness or uncertainty.

3. High intensity of tension, combined with shrinking in length (shortening of shape, stooping, falling), may bring an atmosphere of contained anger in bound flow and uncontrolled temper in free flow. Large amplitudes of such movements, as swooping down, leaping or jumping down, can evoke the image of an attack.

4. Low intensity of tension, combined with growing in length (stretching, rising, straightening), is conducive to easygoing good humor and optimism in free flow and mild

concern in bound flow. When amplitude is low a refinement or delicacy is added.

5. Sudden increases of tension combined with shrinking in depth (hollowing, emptying, withdrawing) in free flow convey preparedness for flight and in bound flow readiness for attack. Angular reversals of direction add a sharp edge to both.

6. Gradual ascent of tension combined with growing in depth (bulging, filling, protruding, approaching), makes for an atmosphere of ponderous but good-natured giving in free flow; in bound flow such an approach takes on the quality of dependability. A curved reversal of directions adds smoothness to the approach.

No one moves in just one combination of movement patterns, but preferred combinations and sequences are characteristic of adult movement and can be detected even in the immature motor patterns of infants. In the kinesthetic interaction between mother and child the affective milieu is created by the propensities of both partners. The mother's preferred motor patterns, mirrored by the child, regulate and modify the child's rhythms. The child's preferred motor patterns evoke positive or negative responses in the mother. In trying to adjust to the child she too begins by mirroring his rhythms to the degree she is capable of doing so. She also anticipates his responses and interprets them as messages before the child is capable of communicating feelings. Her interpretations provide a model for psychic content which the child eventually attaches to the nonverbal transactions between himself and his mother (29).

MATERNAL REACTIONS TO INFANTS' SHAPES

Throughout development, maternal responses to changes in the child's shape organize his flow of shape and provide the atmosphere for successive stages of self-representations, object-representations, and object relationships. In close association with his irregular patterns of breathing, the infant's shape grows and shrinks in an irregular rhythm. In trying to find an order in the bewildering multitude of changes, the mother reacts to predominant changes of shape in the child as if they were expressive of affects familiar to her from previous experiences. Her interpretations of the infant's shapes are influenced by her own predilections as well as by species-determined and learned interpretations of spatial configurations *(11)*. Changes in the conformation of the whole body or its parts (especially head, face, and hands) in combination with appropriate changes in tension-flow become part of nonverbal communication between mother and child.

Growing in width invites contact. Wide shapes inspire confidence even in such small changes as the broadening of the face in integrated smiling *(52)*. In contrast, shrinking in width and narrow shapes, as seen for example in frowning, have a discouraging effect. The most primitive response to narrowing movements is the impulse to make the shrinking object still thinner, to squeeze it until it disappears. But narrow shapes can also evoke pity and a need to enclose them rather than squeeze them. Reaction-formations against the desire to annihilate or ignore the constricted shape and dismiss it as insignificant play a role in the endeavor to nurture and shelter the young. A mother dog selected the runt of her litter to bury in the ground; when it was brought back to her while she nursed the other puppies, she ignored it. Similar reactions occur in young and inexperienced mothers of human infants. Normally however a delicate balance between holding the infant and leaving him alone is not only the result of conflicting maternal emotions but is also due to the changes in the baby's shape from narrowing to widening, from shrinking to growing.

Growing and shrinking in length are taken as communication of intent. In the animal kingdom, growing in the vertical dimension is interpreted as threatening, shrinking as submission. Even facial expressions, such as baring of teeth in which the mouth stretches vertically, are taken as signs of intended attack *(11)*. In man, a slight rising of facial angles conveys elation and 'falling' of features connotes sadness; standing up connotes pride and strength, lying down or falling is identified with surrender. Renouncing one's opposition to gravity or conceding one's inability to cope with it seems to be a model for dejection and defeat *(1)*. A mother may find it difficult to support a tense, stretched-out body and she may become limp and drop it. Consciously or unconsciously afraid that the baby wants to attack her, she may become limp in surrender. When the baby's head falls limply, the usual maternal response is to support it, but some primitive mothers yield to the impulse to drop the small and flaccid, to make it still smaller or ignore it *(10)*.

Growing and shrinking in depth—that is, in the sagittal dimension—connotes action in progress even before locomotion is established. Bulging, protruding into space is associated with satiation, pleasure, fullness, and going ahead. Hollowing is associated with emptiness, hunger, pain, despair, and retreat. The baby's forward movements of head or arms are taken as signs of a positive approach to the mother; the protrusion of his tongue initiates the beginning of appetitive behavior. The neonate's use of his tongue to push out the nipple is a precursor of saying 'stop'. Mothers understand these changes in direction as signals to go ahead or stop the interaction with their babies. They also take them as indications of approval and disapproval on the part of the baby and sometimes react defensively by withdrawing in retaliation or in anticipation of being rejected.

When the child begins to control directions in space, the relation between mother and child becomes less anxiety-laden and more meaningful. Intentional directing of movement in space is a precursor of verbal communication. The formation of words gives meaning to sounds, and sentences shape them into aim-directed vehicles of information. Aim-directed movements such as pointing precede language development, but continue to be the language of movement throughout life. In normal development the mother enjoys each sign of advancement in mastery of communicative interaction. Through her own mature shaping she provides the model for regulation of sequences of approach and withdrawal, and uses changes in shape for the enrichment of her affective relationship with her child.

Space does not permit either a full listing or an exhaustive discussion of the sources of regulation of shape-flow. The following description of stages of this regulation will make reference to the maturing neurophysiological apparatus that come under partial control of the ego. However, its primary theme is the reciprocal regulation of tension-flow and shape-flow, feeling tones and images of self and objects, of efforts and shaping, affective attitudes and transactions with objects in successive stages of object relationships.

THE NARCISSISTIC MILIEU

The mother's adjustment to the infant's tensions and shapes interacts with his own emergent kinesthetic sensations to form the 'narcissistic milieu' (18, 25) of primary identifications from which the child's feelings emerge. These in turn influence and modify tension-flow and shape-flow.

The neonate shudders on hearing loud noises, blinks in 'avoidance' of visual stimuli (30); he is startled in response to sudden changes of his position in relation to gravity (1). He turns toward the source of pleasurable stimuli, be it outward or inward. The kinesthetic responses involved in these reactions are in themselves a source of functional pleasure (8, 18, 28). The more frequent and the more pleasurable the sensations and responses resulting from spontaneous swelling of mucous membranes or from contact with the hand or nipple, the greater tendency there is for movements directed toward the body and the more need to shut out outer stimuli and to inhibit movements toward them.[6]

---

[6] Neonates who suck their own tongues do not react to visual stimuli by turning to them or following with their eyes. But the relationship between reactions to inner and outer stimuli is not always that simple. Wolff and White (53) reported that infants who sucked on pacifiers did not move their heads to follow a visual stimulus but some would move their eyes to do so. In this observation we encounter a harmonious integration of responses to inner and outer stimuli that goes along with centralization of tension-flow and shape-flow, as exemplified in the case of Charlie (30).

High thresholds for external stimuli and lower thresholds for internal stimuli (22), especially from the oral zone, combine with the late maturation of visual and acoustic apparatus to focus the infant's emerging directedness toward his own body. This seems to be the physiological basis for Freud's view that the state of primary narcissism evolves from autoerotism.

The rhythm of shape-flow in the newborn (longer periods and greater frequency of shrinking than growing) facilitates discharge inward, whether the form of discharge is suitable for libido, aggression, or fusions between them (22, 26). The principle of turning away from noxious stimuli is applicable to external stimulation but does not seem to pertain to excitations stemming from the infant's body. Some newborns scratch their faces again and again as if attracted to the source of pain. Colicky infants double up with pain. Discomfort that arises from abdominal sensations interrupts all other activities and the infant's attention seems to center on what is going on inside his body (31). However, the infant's tendency toward discharge inward is counteracted by maturation of apparatus which serve to awaken consciousness. Development brings about an increasing readiness for discharge outward which receives its direction from patterns of maternal care.

The mutuality (16) between mother and child within the narcissistic internal milieu (25) is created by fusion of their body shapes, attunement of their preferred rhythms of tension-flow (30), and harmonizing of their preferred rhythms of shape-flow. Primary identifications are based on transactions in the 'near body space' that belongs to mother and child alike. Mother and child move together, press or touch each other, and are being touched by each other, and in doing so they mirror each other's rhythms and develop feelings for each other. In this type of closeness not only the near space surrounding the body is shared but the 'body space' as well: the infant takes in the nipple and the mother intrudes into his mouth. Within this narrow space of co-functioning (39, 40) there are only a few moments of static unity. Tension-flow and shape-flow change in regular and irregular intervals, one movement evolves from another, and static shapes are kept up in phases of rest, creating a continuum of feeling tones that characterize the milieu in the near space between mother and child.

Two rhythms of alternating union and separation (37) pervade the oral phase of development: 1, a rapidly oscillating rhythm of growing together and shrinking away from each other characterizes the closeness of infant and mother during nursing; 2, being nursed alternates with actual physical separation in two distinct phases of closeness and real distance. After a longer period of separation, fusion in space begins with the child turning to the breast as the mother presents it to him. The sucking rhythm consists of alternating phases of clutching the nipple and releasing it, partially through dropping the jaw (42). This phase of rapidly oscillating minute changes of distance between mother and child ends with the infant releasing the nipple and turning away, which ushers in another long period of separation and a substantial distance is space.

The double periodicity of closeness and distance described here is characteristic of all intimate relationships and all periodic zonal discharge. Through the experience of periodic satisfaction in zonal discharge, shape-flow rhythms differentiate into: 1, zone-specific, multiphasic rhythms that best serve local zonal discharge (30), and 2, bi-phasic rhythms of preparation for zonal discharge by stable, appropriate positioning of the body and return to the shape of rest which terminates contact.

The infant recognizes the nursing position before he has a representation of the object. He learns to turn to the breast (10) and to turn away from it; this gives him a rudiment of control over closeness and distance from the source of satisfaction. This partial independence from the object becomes the core of active initiation and termination of contact according to needs.

REACHING THE ANACLITIC OBJECT

As the child learns the division between phases of preparation, need satisfaction, and termination of contact, head, eye, and hand begin to work in unison. Kinesthetic mirroring of rhythms of tension-flow and shape-flow gradually become supplemented by visually induced mirroring of facial expressions and head and arm movements. Reaching the need-satisfying object develops into a need of its own.

Through attunement of tension and adjustment in shape in the near space between mother and child, they mirror each other's feelings in a reciprocal relationship (39, 40) characteristic of the early oral phase. Guided by the mother's motor patterns, shape-flow differentiates into phases of actions in the service of needs and of reaching the need-satisfying object. Interactions with the need-satisfying object are tinged with feeling tones of comfort and discomfort from which affective self-representations and object-representations differentiate.

Charlie began to smile and coo at five to six weeks. Because of his straining toward her in supine position his mother felt that he was trying to sit up as well. At eight weeks mother proudly exhibited the movement and sound dialogue she and Charlie had been engaging in for some time: 'She talks to him in an excited voice. She touches him and moves her head back and forth and keeps talking, telling him what a good looking fellow he is. He moves his arms toward her; he coos, looks at her intently. Mother moves his legs playfully. He begins to make slight noises of the character of his "drinking" noises. When mother moves he follows with his head. Head, arms, and legs move in slight, slow, medium-amplitude movements.'

The following changes in his movements were stimulated by his mother's mode of excitement: 'Mother tickles his chest and all his limbs move toward her. His mouth opens and closes as if he were in a conversation without sound while his mother talks to him all the time. Mother tells him in a stern voice that he is a bad boy. His face becomes sterner than before. He gestures with face and hands so that one is reminded of a conversation in a silent movie. Mother tells me that he has been "talking" that way for the past three weeks.'

Unfortunately these early recordings do not adequately describe movement patterns. It is apparent, however, that Charlie mirrored the tension and shape of his mother's movements and was beginning to reach out toward her.

Even when he was a neonate Charlie's frame was wide and bulging, which earned him the epithet of 'Churchill'. His shape-flow was conducive to moving sideways and forward which enabled him to carry on this face-to-face communication with his mother, even though she bent her head forward only slightly to meet his eyes. Another infant of two weeks, near his parent's face, mirrored the adult's mouth movements to a remarkable extent. Since this mouth-to-mouth communication was repeated many times, he molded out of it a sound 'hallah' which he began to use instead of crying. This became his 'reach sound' used for calling and greeting during the period between four weeks and four months in which his anaclitic relationships were most prominent.

As the influence of visual and acoustic perceptions increases, kinesthetic and proprioceptive sensations become synesthetically connected with them. Visual representations merge with 'reach' representations to outline objects as separate from the self. In contrast, self-representations, less clearly outlined, never completely differentiate from the shapes of objects perceived in the near body space. In the absence of sight, kinesthetically and acoustically derived shapes of objects are so vividly retained in the child's memory that he may be able to imitate not only shapes and sounds but also facial expressions with amazing accuracy. Burlingham's (9) blind patient, Sylvia, would bend down and tremble as she walked in imitation of her grandmother. She would change her voice when she spoke about her mother or father. When she became attached to the analyst, she began to imitate her facial expressions, smiled as she did, and could reproduce other facial changes. Kinesthetic sensations are closer to feeling tones and can more easily express nonverbal memories than any other sources of representations. Blind children smile in response to voices and touch: the mood intrinsic in the widening of the whole face in integrated smiling, expressed through nonverbal channels of communication, is contagious to the sighted and the blind.[7]

The anaclitic object need not be in the near space of the child as long as it can be reached through movement and through a meeting of moods, based on an attunement and harmony in rhythms of tension-flow and shape-flow. Reaching for an anaclitic object need not be directed; the magic of turning to an external source of satisfaction by movements flowing away from the center of the body, a positioning of limbs, a combination of sounds, may be all the preparation needed to bring the need-satisfying object closer. At first qualities of the object are recognized in the near space in which zonal needs are satisfied. As the infant's horizon expands from the 'near space' through the 'reach space' and into the 'general space', he begins to reach by centrifugal movements directed to the outside. At first he identifies the object by kinesthetically, visually, and acoustically perceived shapes and rhythms familiar to him from experience of close contact. Whereas the anaclitic object is recognized by the 'how' of his movements (tension-flow and shape-flow), the constant object derives its qualities from emergent concepts of 'where, what, and when' (precursors of effort and shaping).

RELATING TO THE CONSTANT OBJECT

The sameness of the object is established by the repetitive character of preferred rhythms of tension-flow and shape-flow, unique to the individual. Memory of the object is based on '. . . the connection of certain moods with the corresponding body sensations which, experienced as one's own body, are transferred onto the other person and then again imitated on one's own body' *(9,* p. 324*)*. The infant recognizes his mother

[7] I am indebted to Mrs. Burlingham for letting me visit the Hampstead Nursery for the Blind, for her many articles and lectures on this subject, and her personal communications. I am also grateful to Miss Wills for allowing me to read the history of a blind child she has observed since infancy.

as distinct from other people because she belongs to his near space and retains these 'near space' qualities in distance transactions as well. In the near space he can feel and smell her, in the reach space he can see her, and in the general space he can either see her or hear her voice. When all these sensory experiences become integrated, the perceived object becomes endowed with a dimensional quality. The relation to the object becomes partially independent from zonal needs and more and more guided by mastery of spatial directions, which all converge in the narrow sector of space in which the object reappears. In successive developmental stages, intentional directing of movement regulates shape-flow in accordance with dominant needs that mold the relationship to objects: primarily sideways and across in the oral stage, primarily up and down in the anal stage, and primarily forward and backward in the urethral stage. As self-representations and object-representations become multidimensional, they become endowed with qualities related to space, weight, and time, and feelings toward the constant object gain in scope, intensity, and depth.

Through reaching out into wider and more varied realms of space, the changing shapes of the body effect a change in the gestalt of space, as they divide it into large and small sections by lines and loops, sharp angles and smooth curves. Fleeting 'shaping' of space by spreading or enclosing, rising or descending, advancing or retiring, corresponds to fleeting fantasies which begin to organize feelings toward objects. In the early 'inner-genital' stage which precedes phallic development, pregenital drives become integrated with 'genital' urges (31). Trying to escape from internal sensations the child externalizes them to outside objects, becomes outward-directed, and deliberately imitative. He identifies with his mother and actively reproduces her motor patterns. He builds play configurations concretely to represent fantasies about the 'inner space' inside his body and that of his mother (15). In the phallic phase, the child's total body is sexualized and outer space is identified with his love object whom he seeks to penetrate as a whole. In atency, the child subordinates rhythms of tension-flow to 'efforts' and rhythms of shape-flow to 'shaping' of space in accordance with socially acceptable requirements of work and play. Not until adolescence does he consistently use all elements of effort and all planes of space at once in postures and gestures. He begins to perform like an adult in work and sports, but his conflicts in relation to objects are expressed in contradictory shaping so that his posture may be inviting and the simultaneous or ensuing gesture may be rejecting. Object relationships of adults are expressed in harmonious movements in which shaping of space subordinates rhythms of shape-flow in various parts of the body to best serve as a vehicle for feelings and attitudes carried by ego-controlled tension-flow and effort. The constancy of adult relationships is reflected in the constancy of preferred phases of effort-shape combinations—in gestures and postures—that characterize permanent movement profiles (32, 36). The manner in which adults express their personalities through movement is predicated on congenital preferences for certain patterns of movement and their modifications in successive stages of drive and ego development.

THE ROLE OF THE HORIZONTAL PLANE IN THE ORAL PHASE

In the oral phase, communication between mother and child occurs primarily in the 'feeding' or 'table plane' (4, 34, 36, 41, 44, 45). The infant conveys acceptance or rejection through precursors of shaping in the horizontal plane which remains the plane of communication throughout life.

In the oral phase, reaching becomes preparatory for seizing and taking. Shape-flow is then organized in phases of growing to reach, local shrinking to scoop, and further shrinking to take in. At the same time the object becomes endowed with constancy of spatial qualities. Near or far, away from the body or in it, the object belongs to a space the child has made his own. In the early oral phase, turning to the object in the near body sphere brings about a meeting and fusing of body shapes; the totality of object representations is based on a feeling of growing together and merging rhythms of tension-flow and shape-flow. In the oral-sadistic stage, directing of movements toward the object is a preparation for seizing, clutching, and incorporating. These transactions occur primarily in the two dimensions of the table or feeding plane: the principal dimension of the horizontal plane is sideways-across and its accessory dimension, forward and backward.

Scanning of the horizon helps the child to find the object. Moving sideways, right and left, and seeking in free-floating attention, he changes levels of intensity of tension and he widens, traversing a sinuous pathway with head and arms. These are precursors of an indirect approach to space through 'efforts', of directional 'shaping' sideways, and of spreading in both dimensions of the horizontal plane. Once the child finds the object and localizes it, his attention becomes bound, the level of tension stabilizes, and he narrows in a linear movement. These are precursors of a direct approach to space through 'effort', of directional 'shaping' across, and enclosing space in both dimensions of the horizontal plane. His feeling during scanning might be, 'Is it here, is it there?'; when he channels his attention to a focal point, he may feel, 'It is there'. He turns to it, cathects it, smiles, reaches for it, and makes it his own. When he refuses to cathect it, he turns away from it, cannot see it any more: 'It is not there'. The persistence of the constant object is based on acceptance of the existence of the real object in space.

As attention becomes channeled, the tension bound and its level even, the oral rhythm too changes in quality. The oscillating sucking rhythm no longer shows soft transitions from free to bound flow and vice versa; holding the nipple with even bound flow and biting on it becomes more frequent (30, 31). Free and bound flow reverse sharply and linear movements change directions in angles. Kinesthetic sensations of channeled, linear, and sharp movements help to outline more clearly the shape of self-representations and object-representations.

With more frequent feeding of solids to the child in an

upright position, a reciprocal relation develops between mother and child in which activity and passivity take on a rhythmic quality *(37)*. Distance feeding makes the horizontal plane (table plane) more meaningful to the child. He becomes more aware of his mother's feeding movements which change direction from forward-across to backward-sideways. He mirrors her movements without yet understanding the significance of directions in space. Soon he begins to feed himself and generously gives some food to his mother also. The give-and-take interplay becomes the basis for his relation to his mother. Refusal and withdrawal are reserved for the stranger *(50, 51)* whose shape and rhythms of shape-flow are unfamiliar and whose mood is alien too as he intrudes into the space between mother and child and distorts it by his intrusion. The child may reconcile himself with the stranger if careful study of his features and demeanor allows him to perceive tensions, shapes, and feeling tones similar to his own. At times, however, as familiar a person as his mother may appear strange when her mood changes unexpectedly or when her shape alters in an unaccustomed dimension (for example, by the addition of a hat or a large piece of fur).

In the early phase of object constancy, acceptance is based on recognition of sameness, and rejection on clashing with dissimilarities. Acceptance is conveyed by a broad smile, rejection by a stern or anxious face. Reaching and taking are operations which imply acceptance. Turning to the side and backward when an unaccepted object draws closer is a precursor of refusal in a 'no' gesture.

In previous papers I described how Charlie clashed with his mother because of discrepancies in their rhythms of tension-flow *(29, 30)*. The following description of Charlie's difficulties will focus on the importance of appropriate planes and directions in feeding.

At seven months, Charlie had refused solids and had stopped reaching for objects. But he regularly smiled at his mother even when quite uncomfortable because of teething pain. He stared at me for a long time before he gave me a smile. He did not reject his mother; he rejected, so to speak, his feeding mother. It was impressive to watch the determination with which he refused the spoonfuls she handed to him. She stood up in front of a low table at which Charlie sat slumping down and forward. When the spoon reached his mouth from above, he spat and turned his head sideways and backward. He could not see his mother as she would not stoop and he could not look up. The spoon seemed to follow him when he turned away and once again Charlie turned away from it, backward and sideways in the opposite direction, and cried. He could enjoy feeding when one sat down at his eye level and he could participate actively in coming forward to the spoon.

Even though Charlie got over his crisis of feeding and reaching, he retained the difficulty in communicating with his mother in certain situations and clashed in a similar manner with his teachers. I remember vividly a scene during his latency which appeared to be a replica of his early refusal to eat. Mother asked him an arithmetic question. She stood in her habitual shape of imminent retreat, her trunk slightly hollow, her head bent forward a bit but not directed down enough to meet the gaze of the child. Charlie stood in front of her, looking forward and down and veering sideways. His dazed look, familiar to me from his infancy, made it very clear that he could not think. Then, as in his infancy, when I sat down with him and established a face-to-face communication in the horizontal plane, he could reach out for help; with some direction he started to think on his own and triumphantly produced the right answer.

THE ROLE OF THE VERTICAL PLANE IN THE ANAL PHASE

In the oral phase, the child communicates the state of his needs by acceptance or rejection. In the anal phase he learns to present his intent or feelings in relation to objects. He shows the manner in which he appraises himself and others through precursors of shaping in the vertical plane. This plane remains the plane of presentation throughout life (4, 35, 36).

In the anal phase, holding and relinquishing divides the rhythm of shape-flow into prolonged shrinking while holding, and brief growing-out into space while releasing or throwing. At this time the child gains control over degrees of tension. At first he may keep the tension at the same level of intensity or lower it. The sphincter becomes the focal point for these alterations in degree of tension, control of which is a precursor of the 'effort' of lightness. In the anal-sadistic phase the child gains control over higher degrees of tension, the precursor of the 'effort' of strength. He presses hard with his abdominal muscles and contracts his sphincter with determination; at the same time he begins to control antigravity muscles through his whole body. As he stands up, the vertical plane of his body begins to conform to the vertical plane of space—the wall-plane or door-plane *(41, 44, 45)*. As he gets up and lets himself down, he becomes familiar with the principal dimension of the vertical plane. When he throws things, he moves down and sideways or across; when he lifts things high, he moves up and sideways or across. Thus he gets the feeling of both dimensions of the vertical plane. He becomes acquainted with the qualities of heavy and light, strong and weak by the extent to which he can lift or lower things. The apparatus of spatial 'weighing' and comparing small and big, light and heavy, weak and strong facilitates the persistence of object constancy despite ambivalence of feelings: big and remote, small and easy, strong and hostile, light and gentle, up or down, rising or descending, the self and the object retain their identity. As the child begins to hold back and release intentionally, he becomes aware of intent in himself and others. But mothers often organize shape and directions before the child can understand them or initiate them himself. They guide innate responses to tensing and releasing, shrinking and growing in the vertical dimension by attaching positive and negative values to them.

At seven months, Charlie was taught the game 'so big'. His mother would initiate it by saying 'so big' with great glee and stretching the child's arm upward. Charlie might respond by raising his knees, but soon he would follow with up-and-down movements, accompanied by intense straining with appropriate sounds. At that time Charlie responded with controlled tension-flow and shape-flow; he could not yet control the vertical dimension of his body. Months later, he would raise himself up proudly and lift toys for his mother to see; he would point to a chair persistently with imperious downward gestures to indicate that his mother must sit down on it. Earlier he had expressed his discontent with the results of her erectness by refusing food; at that time he could accept or reject but could not formulate his intent as he could now. When he accepted his mother's sense of values and was proud of being 'so big' and erect himself, his self-importance gave him the prerogative of imposing his wishes upon his mother in an unequivocal way. Because he could convey his intent with authority and determination, she listened to him and would sit down at his request.

As the child becomes proficient in getting up and stooping down, his feelings of self evolve from cognizance of his whole extended body and his budding recognition that he has a center of gravity and can shift it. As he begins to control the defecation rhythm (30), he prepares himself for defecation by squatting. He likes this position and will squat while playing. Maintaining this body shape, he controls things on the floor; he throws them and retrieves them at will. As he becomes bolder, the amplitude of his movements grows. As he feels his own weight and compares it with the little, light things he can dominate, he begins to 'throw his weight around'. His wish becomes law; opposition to his will provokes fights and temper. When he wins he feels big and when he loses he feels small.

Surrounded by many things that are easy to locate and reach, he is busy selecting and discarding. But he is not always determined; he begins to question and doubt. He changes from high to low intensity of tension, from large to small in size, from rising to letting himself down. His feeling tones change from high to low spirits, from pride to despair. His relationship to objects becomes highly ambivalent. His approval of himself and objects becomes reciprocal in the sense that he is big when they are small and vice versa. As his aggression increases, he begins to struggle to maintain his self-representation as a contained functioning unit despite variations of shapes and feelings. The same struggle for retaining the image of the object despite its changing moods and shapes imbues the relationship to his mother. She may be threatening and unyielding, towering over him, or friendly, stooping down to him, picking him up, and submitting to his will. Through all these changes in shape and mood on his part and hers, she retains the unique quality of being his mother. She becomes his sparring partner. He contends with her and craves her, and expects her presence.

In the first stage of constancy the object was 'there' or 'not there', depending on the child's acceptance or rejection. Then the permanent qualities of the object become established and the object becomes 'that' person and not another. Once the mother remains the same despite some changes in her attributes, the child can afford to send his mother away and to retrieve her at will (22). Because the core of her representation remains constant, he can show her his anger without fear. He can idealize her or despise her by looking up to her or looking down on her. He can accept her or reject her, approve of her or condemn her; but not before he becomes proficient in walking can he put plans into operation that carry out any of his intents with efficiency. When he was creeping, he began to leave her and come back to her; at that time he needed only to look up and back to find her. When he walks away from her the danger of losing her is greater. As he is involved in weighing and appraising, his ambivalence, expressed in the up-and-down qualities of his movements, makes it difficult for him to decide what to do.

THE ROLE OF THE SAGITTAL PLANE IN THE URETHRAL PHASE

Although anal and urethral interests overlap, the distinction between the predominant rhythms, shapes, and preferred directions in anal and urethral zonal activities suggest a division into two separate developmental stages (31).

In the urethral phase, the child begins to put decisions into operation. He moves forward and backward in the sagittal plane which remains the plane of operational transaction throughout life (35, 36). Running to and away from objects preserves the continuity of self and objects in time and space. Conversely, the continuity of object-representations allows for self-reliance in exploration of space for longer periods of time.

As the child gains control over the urinary stream, he turns from passive surrender to the flow of urine to active holding back, releasing it and directing it. He begins to raise and lower intentionally the rate of increase and decrease of tension. This control is a precursor of the 'efforts' of acceleration and deceleration. The child deliberately bulges and directs the stream of urine forward and downward, 'hollows' again at the end of urination, and retreats. As he stops and goes, he uses precursors of shaping forward or backward, downward or upward which are the principal and accessory dimensions of the sagittal plane. At the same time that he learns to control his position for urination and gains control over the urinary stream, he also begins to master spatial directions and continuity and discontinuity in locomotion. 'Stop' and 'go' become important transactions between himself and his mother. His right to initiate suddenly or gradually, to continue or interrupt, becomes very precious to him. As he begins to appreciate his own continuity in time despite intervals of discontinuity in movement, he also becomes confident that he will always find his mother. The image of his mother is there, unchanging, not only in the near space, not only in the reach space, but also in the general space into which he ventures. He becomes an expert operator: he decides when to start or stop, when to lead, when to follow, when to run away, and when to turn back. These decisions control his mother's movements if she does not want to lose sight of him. She has to follow him, but even if she lags behind he is confident that she will reappear. The constant object becomes enriched by its new quality of continuity in time. Doing things is so important now that it can bridge the gap of time and make intervals of mother's absence seem shorter. Operations are divided by going away from mother and returning to bring her tangible evidence of exploits. The child becomes enamored of the feeling of mastery over advance and retreat in the sagittal dimension. He not only goes forward and backward himself at will but he makes things come to him, follow him or go away from him as he pleases. The magic of volitional and controlled advance and propelling forward, retreat and pushing back, includes the world of animate and inanimate objects.

INSIDE AND OUTSIDE IN THE 'INNER GENITAL' PHASE

The child between two-and-a-half and four who has achieved a good deal of mastery over his pregenital drives has learned to apply specific rhythms of tension-flow and shape-flow and specific preparatory positioning for the satisfaction of zonal needs. He becomes able to select rhythms of tension-flow and shape-flow as well as their attributes in the service of functions. In nonzonal activities he uses a great many modified rhythms; at first divergent rhythms may jar with each other but gradually an integration of pregenital rhythms is accomplished. One can note the influence of a special rhythm of tension-flow that helps to combine the previously described rhythms into integrated sequences. This rhythm, I believe, serves the discharge of genital drives whose source is in the inside of the body (such as vagina or spermatic cords). It consists of prolonged phases of gradually ascending free flow that change equally gradually into bound flow. Combined with softly changing directions which design waves in space, this type of rhythm gives the three-year old a quality of poise that resolves the disequilibrium of the two-and-a-half-year old *(31)*. This rhythm is particularly suitable for spreading of inner sensations all over the body and outside of it through externalization.

The precedipal child stages games in which he identifies with his mother's planned motor activity. He imitates what she is doing in the setting of a play that has a beginning, a theme, and an end. His sentences become grammatical and his movements assume structure. He chooses a direction, makes fleeting designs in space, and changes direction again. He begins to move in diagonals that traverse space in all directions at once—forward-sideways-down, for example. Division of space by diagonals is a necessary prerequisite for the understanding of multidimensionality and differentiation between the inside and outside of objects. The child erects walls with blocks in a manner showing his recognition of planes that divide the inside space, enclosed by walls, from outer space. His buildings are becoming three dimensional; things are narrow or wide, tall or short, fat or thin, filled or empty. Using some fleeting 'efforts' and some precursors of 'effort', the child can now direct his attention to space, weight, and time all at once. He can say: '*Now* I pick *up* a *heavy* block', and do it.

From the midst of even flow that he uses to maintain precision, there arise moments of directness, expressive of his ability to stick to a point for a short while. He can become indirect by changing from plane to plane but he cannot follow through to completion (he can twist but not yet knot). He picks up heavy objects mostly by high intensity of bound flow of tension but glimpses of real strength can be seen too. He does not often use strength, but in dealing with small articles he employs lightness rather than just low intensity of tension. He controls the rate of increase and decrease of tension and begins to understand the temporal effect of his fleeting accelerations and decelerations.

As the child is becoming skilful in controlling attributes of tension-flow, his affective repertoire increases. This can be noted in his facial expressions, the intonation of his speech, and his beginning gesticulation. He is becoming more proficient in using small excursions of movement instead of much larger ones, in reversing directions sharply or softly. But in excitement he jumps every which-way, as various parts of his body move in uncoördinated rhythms of tension-flow and shape-flow.

The beginning multidimensional approach of the child at this stage gives him some understanding of the 'inside space' in himself and others. By externalization into outer space and to the periphery of his body, he forms concepts about 'inside' shapes. He arranges things in relation to one another, organizing their configurations in space by imitation of his mother's real activities and those he imagines her to be engaged in. He identifies with her and stages games in which he plays her part. But his father is becoming more and more important; the child imitates masculine characteristics too and divides shapes of the body and qualities of movement into male and female categories. Men become identified for him with protrusion in space, with strength and speed, with spreading, ascending, and advancing in space. Women are endowed with the opposite attributes. Men are conceived as tall, arrowlike, and solid; women as enclosed and hollow 'inside'. The confined space of the home is recognized as the domain of the mother; father deals with the general space coveted by the child. Toward the end of this phase, inner genital sensations are externalized to the periphery of the body, thus accentuating body boundaries. Rejection of the 'inside' space brings on a hypercathexis of the phallic body and the outer space.

THE OUTER SPACE IN THE PHALLIC PHASE

In the phallic phase, the whole solid body becomes sexualized as it gets into the service of 'completely object centered phallic-oedipal' *(18)* relationships. All parts of the body acting synchronously create definite designs in space in correspondence with fantasies about self and objects *(12, 13, 14, 15, 16)*. This type of movement is a precursor of postural shaping.

The child in the phallic phase leaps, jumps, and swings in coördinated rhythms of tension-flow and shape-flow. His favored rhythm of tension-flow is an alternation between small intensities of bound flow and abruptly ascending and descending high intensities of free flow (30). His shape-flow tends to alternate between low amplitudes in shortening and high amplitudes in lengthening and protruding. He likes moving upward and forward but he also enjoys falling down and sliding backward. His whole body participates in these extreme changes which are well suited to his rhythm of activity and passivity: penetrating and being penetrated (16). He goes from intense wooing to rejection and annihilation of the object, from active conquering to passive surrender, from grandiose attacks to anxious expectations of counterattacks. These are dressed in elaborate fantasies in which designs in space play a major role. He races, flies, and explodes into space or surrenders with pleasure to being tossed around and whirled about. He becomes a 'space addict'; he not only dreams of traversing it in lines and loops, high up and crashing down, in sharp angles and soft spiral waves, but he also experiments with space through acrobatic stunts. The phallic child identifies space with his love object. He wants to get into it, fill it, and conquer it; he wants to be engulfed in it, carried by it, and surrender to it. But he dreams more than he can do.

Although he uses his whole body in abundance, his efforts and shaping do not yet control his tension-flow and shape-flow. On the contrary, his effort and shaping patterns are subservient to his preferred rhythms. He cannot coördinate efforts and shapes too well, nor can he follow through with the same effort-shape pattern when he moves his whole body in a unified rhythm of tension-flow and shape-flow (precursor of postures). An undue amount of free flow may derail his adaptive movement so that he can easily hurt himself or others in the exercise of his bold adventures in space. Out of sheer love he can 'squeeze to death' as the deceleration and lightness of loving embrace deteriorates into high intensity of tension and acceleration; he can pull people down as he hugs them by being derailed from the horizontal to the vertical plane. Conversely, in attacking his enemy with strength he may suddenly lapse into free flow and lightness; trying to jump him, he may jump so high in preparation that he misses his aim and falls flat on his face.

CONSOLIDATION OF EFFORT AND SHAPE IN LATENCY

In latency, regulation of tension-flow by 'efforts' and of shape-flow by 'shaping' becomes consolidated to the extent that the reasonable ego gains control over unbridled fantasies and diffuse feelings. Consonance of movement is achieved through coördination of aim-directed efforts and shaping of spatial configurations that best serve the aim.

A latency child is capable of using strength and acceleration in hammering. Soon he finds out that he will do a better job if he shapes his movements in such a way that his arm descends and advances toward the nail he tries to hammer in. He is not simply stretching the arm forward and down as he would in reaching or pointing. He traverses the principal and the accessory dimensions of the vertical and sagittal planes as he moves from sideways-backward-high to forward-low and across. He uses the principal dimension of the vertical plane going down and the accessory dimension by turning across; he uses the principal dimension of the sagittal plane as he advances and its accessory dimension as he comes down. The direction 'down' is emphasized in this example because it belongs to both planes. But were the child to use it merely as a direction instead of shaping in planes, he would lose either strength or speed and his work movement would become less efficient.

As the superego develops, a systemization of values causes division of work from play. The child learns a great many skills through imitation of adults and explanations of techniques. Without a model for a well-integrated motor pattern he uses fewer effort-shape combinations, just as he can tell a familiar story fairly well but when he creates his own stories the sentences and their sequence do not clearly express what he wants to convey. The coördination between content (effort) and form (shaping) is in its beginnings; the child is learning to find an adequate structure for expressing himself and he does so by

imitation and by conforming to self-imposed rules and standards of adults and peers. When he is guided by rules of games
and aims of work, he subordinates rhythms of tension-flow and
shape-flow to 'efforts' and 'shaping' of movement in space. However, even under well-regulated conditions he is rarely able to
take all the factors of motion into consideration at once. He
rarely exhibits well-coördinated motor patterns in postural
movements. His attitudes are not yet well defined. His concepts
of space, weight, and time are limited and his relationships are
determined by the standards of family and school. He cannot
yet make substantial changes in the world around him although he has achieved a measure of autonomy so that he can
proceed on his own in small matters. Correspondingly, he uses
integrated effort-shape patterns primarily in gestures and rarely
in postures.

PROGRESSION AND REGRESSION IN ADOLESCENCE

The most conspicuous progress in adolescence is due to the
maturation of apparatus which help to objectivize space, weight,
and time. Concepts of the forces of nature become independent
of object relations. At the same time, the maturing concrete and
abstract knowledge of spatial relations aids the adolescent in
finding new ways of relating to people. His skills in sports and
work increase rapidly as does his ability to participate in team
work. His interests and communications encompass many subjects and his compositions, in writing, speaking, or movement,
become more meaningful and better organized. But he is not
as steady as he was in latency when his skills were fewer but
his performance was more dependable and his controls less
reversible.

As the adolescent develops independent adaptive attitudes
to space, weight, and time, he also becomes totally involved in
interactions with people and in goal-directed tasks. Correspondingly, he can use three 'efforts' and/or 'shape' elements in one
action—not only in gestures but also in postures (as required
for effective punching, hammering, pitching, etc.). But he

frequently expresses his conflicts by a discrepancy between 'effort' or 'shape' elements in gestures and postures. Exaggerations of stylized postural shaping may be unexpectedly followed by an awkward gesture in which neither direction nor design conforms to the preceding effort-shape pattern. There is a great contrast in his behavior in states of high and low motivation. These states change in accordance with alterations in quantity and quality of drive impulses, and in correspondence with fluctuations in goal directedness.

The adolescent's ability to use his whole body effectively reflects the cohesiveness of the synthetic function of his ego and the greater awareness of his own identity within a group. However, his self-image undergoes changes and so does the shape of his body; this occurs not only because of alterations in actual size and body contours but also because of shifting identifications which affect carriage, gait, and relations of limbs to each other. He is subject to rapid disorganization when his motivation to perform decreases or an onrush of drive impulses breaks down the synthetic function in such a way that a diffusion of feelings blurs his newly found identity. He may then lose control over rhythms of tension-flow and shape-flow; various rhythms may compete with each other, and some parts of the body move one way while others exhibit contrasting qualities of movement. As he spreads into the surrounding space in free flow, his shape grows markedly but this impression is belied by the shrinking in his tight fists or by the twisting of his toes.

It is interesting to watch the contrast of early adolescent movement during a dance class and during a recess.[8] While dancing the youngsters can execute a series of phrases of movement in which all motion factors combine to express their feelings, attitudes, and aspirations in harmonious postures and matching gestures. Alone or in groups they seem capable of relating to space, gravity, and time with appropriate rhythms of tension-flow and shape-flow, with definite effort-shape com-

8 I am grateful to Lillian Harmel of London for letting me notate movement patterns during dance classes of different age groups.

binations and graceful transitions from one movement pattern to another. In contrast, during recess they fall all over each other in disorganized rhythms and inappropriate efforts and shapes, in a series of gestures whose imbalance expresses a chaotic disintegration of self-images, object-representations and relationships. This difference in motor behavior reflects the wide range between progression and regression characteristic of adolescents.

Through countless regressions and progressions of drive and ego organization, a redistribution of cathexes creates a new order which brings about a permanent shape and a harmonious effort-shape repertoire in the postures and gestures of the adult.

ADULT CONSTANCY

Adult harmony of movement is an indicator of harmony in the ego which comes about when the ego successfully mediates between the demands of id, superego, the ego's own interests, and the demands of the outside world (7). The adult movement profile is a fine measure of the degree and nature of the ego's success or failure in achieving harmony.

In optimal adjustment, adults control tension-flow, reserving appropriate rhythms for specific zonal and functional discharge and mingling pure zonal, merged, and modified rhythms in various sequences for the expression of affects. Through attunement with sexual partners they evolve adult genital rhythms that are suitable for mutual satisfaction and yet retain characteristics unique to the individual. Through control of shape-flow, adults become capable of expressing moods, feelings, and finer shades of relating to people. Tendencies toward certain static shapes of the body (wide or narrow, elongated or short, bulging or hollow, straight or twisted, angular or soft) from which shaping of the surrounding space evolves, reflect adult concepts of self which influence the style of relationships. Typical combinations of 'effort' and 'shaping' patterns outline individual ranges of adjustment to the forces of nature and the world of objects. To the degree that these combinations or single elements are the same in postures as in gestures, we can appraise the area of the adult's conflict-free functioning. In studying the discrepancies between movement patterns used in postures and gestures, we can gain insight into the nature of conflicts and modes of defense mechanisms characteristic of an individual.

The constancy of individual character traits is expressed in the permanently established preferences for certain 'effort' elements and their combinations. The constancy of individual modes of relating to objects is expressed in the permanently established preferences for certain styles of 'shaping'.

'Efforts' are the dynamic factors of movement, through which various degrees and combinations of aggression and libido are dispensed by the ego to create an impact on the environment. As they control tension-flow they tame drive expressions and serve defenses against drives; in their control of the environment they serve adaptation to reality. Efforts alone cannot make an impact unless they are organized through 'shaping', directed by the ego in accordance with culturally acceptable modes of behavior dictated by the taste of an era *(35, 36)*. Efforts can be compared with words and shaping with sentence structure through which we convey meaningful messages. Efforts without shape lack structure, shapes without effort are empty, devoid of content. Shaping of space alone conveys form but as a vehicle for efforts it expresses object-related ideas, feelings, yearnings, ideals, aspirations, and conflicts and their resolution.

It is likely that directness in approaching space, increase in strength, and acceleration serve aggressive motor discharge controlled by the ego. There is an affinity between these patterns and shaping in concave movements of enclosing, descending, and retreating. Indirectness in approaching space, lightness, and deceleration are likely to denote attitudes of indulgence which serve ego controlled discharge of libido. There is an affinity between these patterns and shaping in convex movements of spreading, rising, and advancing. This rough classification does not do justice to the variety of attitudes toward objects that shaping in space can convey. Furthermore, the six elements of effort and the six elements of shape combine in many different ways and in various sequences. In addition, various combinations of tension-flow and shape-flow, alone or in conjunction with efforts and shaping, bring an even greater complexity into phrases of movement.

The simplest type of shaping is directional, toward or away from the body in the three dimensions of space. Shapes thus created convey approach to or withdrawal from a given point in space. From changes of shape-flow—wide to narrow, big to small, bulging to hollow, and vice versa—there evolve directed movements which are used as preparations for more complex shaping of space between self and objects. Shaping in directions initiates or maintains a relationship; shaping in planes conveys the themes in the interaction between people.

In the horizontal plane, we invite or terminate contact and convey how our attention is directed toward objects. We enclose a narrow segment of space to narrow down an issue or to pay attention to one person to whom we direct our efforts. By spreading over a larger area of space, we prepare for a flexible, indirect approach for which we must be ready to move from one plane to another. Transactions in the horizontal plane serve communication (35, 36) of ideas, plans, and suggestions, as well as acceptance or rejection of thoughts expressed by others.

In the vertical plane we present our intent, our feelings about ourselves and others, our wishes and convictions (35, 36). We rise as we show qualities of leadership, and we descend as we yield. But when we feel strongly about a matter we 'put our foot down', and feeling lighthearted we may wave our hand upward and sideways. We express doubt by alternating between rising and descending, and we frequently do so by raising an eyebrow or by rhythmic alternations between downward and upward motions of head or hand from right to left and left to right. We may even design a question mark in space by appropriate shaping in the vertical plane.

In the sagittal plane we put our intent into operation. We

deal in it with progression in time, with quickness of decision, slowing down of transactions, or wavering between acceleration and deceleration, between advance and retreat (35, 36). Approach in the horizontal plane has the nature of clinging or seeking; in the sagittal plane we approach people to follow them or invite them to follow us. In the horizontal plane withdrawal conveys rejection; in the sagittal plane it may indicate retreating or inviting a change in the direction of the operation.

As we change from plane to plane, change directions, or move in three directions all at once through diagonal movements, our body shape changes to facilitate shaping of space. We create configurations in the surrounding space designed to influence the spectator. In painting the artist can reproduce a shape, the relation of its parts to each other, and even the change in the gestalt of the surrounding space by the way he captures the latent movement in the static design of body shape and spatial configurations. The three-dimensional quality of sculpture can better express how space is altered by the shape of bodies, but only dance can convey a succession of themes through the changing qualities of space between mover and spectator.

In studying rhythms of shape-flow from which shaping evolves, we begin to get a glimpse of the scope of affective interactions between objects. From the habitually preferred static shapes and the flow of shape in movement and from shaping in spatial planes and directions we hope to gain insight into the way permanent and fluctuating images of self and object create the affective milieu of nonverbal communication. We can appraise the contradictory messages people give and receive from the way one part of the body moves in one pattern while another simultaneously or successively distorts the former (6, 36). If the motor patterns used in gestures are vastly different from those used in postures, it indicates a failure of the ego to maintain harmony between functioning in states of low motivation and in states of high motivation. Lack of harmony between certain patterns of tension-flow and shape-flow, of efforts and shaping, reflects the failure of the ego in coördinating drive expressions and adaptive functioning in relation to objects. The widening of the face in a smile becomes a grin when it combines with a high degree of bound flow *(33)*; 'putting one's foot down' lightly is an empty gesture in which we recognize that the mover has no real intent to assert himself and only tries to give the appearance of doing so.

In an introductory presentation of new concepts, it is difficult to steer between the perils of oversimplification and lack of clarity. Brief reports of harmonizing and clashing relationships in three mother-child pairs may show the complexity of psychological assessment derived from motor profiles; they may also clarify issues left obscure in the text.

The following reports are excerpts from longitudinal studies of three children who have been observed periodically since birth. They are now twelve-and-a-half years old *(29, 30)*.

Glenda's persistent preference for suddenly erupting and suddenly waning free flow, combined with a long and narrow shape of her body, from which further growing in length emerges, conveys her enthusiasm and optimism. But her affect is spent quickly, and her narrowness restricts contact. Her mother's wide shape as well as her gradual ascent of tension and controlled fluctuations of degree of tension convey warmth and readiness to adjust to the child's needs.

Although mother and child move lightly, Glenda appears springy and lighter than she may really be because of her frequent rising and stressing the upward direction; her mother seems heavier than she actually is because she tends to sink and rarely moves upward. Glenda accelerates and advances, giving the impression of rushing but this tendency is well balanced by richness in downward shaping which, so to speak, keeps her feet on the ground. Her mother spreads in the horizontal plane but is not as flexible as this seems to indicate. Her preference for deceleration and her fair ability to accelerate are poorly matched by rare advancing and even less frequent retreating in the sagittal plane.

In postural movements, Glenda displays many attributes

learned from her mother: gradual ascent of tension and controlled flow fluctuations, especially in low intensity. But in contrast to her mother who becomes bound in postures, Glenda's free flow increases even more when she is totally involved. Both mother and daughter become more indirect and use more strength and downward shaping in postural movements. Even though indirect in their approach, they can become determined and forceful so that there is a contest of wills between them when they disagree and a contagious increase of intent when they do agree. But, throughout this, Glenda remains free and easy while her mother becomes overconcerned and worried.

Glenda's relatively rare use of directness and horizontal shaping results in insufficient exploration of ideas and poor focusing on a plan of action. When her intent becomes strong enough she rushes forth carrying out projects that are not well thought out. Her mother can communicate better and brings up issues for consideration. But her many flow fluctuations and wide spreading, her deceleration and her relatively rare use of advance or retreat are reflected in her rambling and her indecisiveness. When she is upset she can give orders with authority, but her great excitement and her tendency to become rigid and repetitive, yet indirect, interfere with a clear presentation of intent. She wavers between strength and lightness, between deceleration and acceleration, while at the same time she tends to become immobilized by boundness and a lack of decision whether to advance or retreat. It seems that she is unable to cope with problems effectively when her aggression increases. In contrast, Glenda's wishes become very clear and she quickly decides what to do and goes ahead with it. Although she does not come forth with a plan herself, she can organize many operations that her mother would not be able to carry out without her help.

The milieu of warmth and acceptance that emerges from the mother meets the child's enthusiasm with a mixture of pride, approval, and anxious concern. Throughout a visit one can observe adjustment to mood changes, encouragement or ambivalent scolding that inhibits the child or slows her down.

Occasionally one gets a glimpse of strong disciplinary measures. It is interesting to note that this combination provides a benign climate for the child's exhibiting what mother and child both strive for but which mother has too much conflict to achieve for herself. The interaction between mother and child encourages the latter to carry out progressive fulfilments of ambition which are beyond the mother's ability to organize. Mother's pride in her daughter's achievement is marred only by her own anxiety, but she is always gratified because Glenda's bold manner in coping with situations as they arise belies her maternal concern.

Nancy's permanently established narrow shape only rarely permits movement venturing beyond her near space. Shrinking, and thus drawing still closer to herself, occurs four times as often as growing, and the latter is confined to small amplitudes. With beginning adolescence Nancy lost some of the extreme rigidity she used to display and has become more lively. Her tension-flow approximates her mother's when she is in her mother's presence. This is probably due to a persistence of mirroring.

Both mother and Nancy use very few postural movements and rarely shape in planes. Both tend to accelerate, and neither uses strength. The mother's preference for downward, across, and forward directions results in her missing contact with Nancy who preferably moves upward and retreats. There is no real communication between them. Nancy still operates with even tension-flow instead of directness, and her narrowness prevents her from moving horizontally.

Nancy's inability to reach directly for what is offered interferes with development of identifications that are usually operative in transactions with people. Even when Nancy does reach out sometimes, she is unable to take in and receive but she shrinks and hollows instead. Her behavior is reminiscent of her infancy when she could not grasp a toy but went after the hand that held it (30). A conversation with Nancy is possible only by an unceasing effort of the interviewer and the mother's demand that she respond. In those rare moments when Nancy's motivation increases, she uses exclusively 'fighting' efforts (directness, strength, or acceleration); these create very little impact because her movements, directed upward and forward, give the illusion of shadow-boxing.

Mother and child are anaclitically oriented, but Nancy is much closer to the stage of transition from narcissism to anaclitic clinging. Maturation of efforts and directional shaping have given her tools for performing in a world of hazy self-images and object-representatives. She seems to progress by mirroring rather than by identification with objects.

Although each of the three children changed through the years of observation (29, 30), beginning adolescence accentuated alterations in movement patterns in Charlie more than in the others. Nevertheless, one can trace the links between his present attitudes and his behavior in infancy.

Charlie's wide and bulging frame persisted through early latency, but gave way to a narrow and more elongated shape with the approach of adolescence. His original preference for gradual emergence of tension still persists but he is now quite capable of displaying sudden eruptions of tension. This seems to be the result of his adjustment to his family's rhythms of tension-flow, but it is now accentuated by the increased urgency of his drives. Even more striking is the change from habitual deceleration to a preference for acceleration. His tendency to direct his movements downward is still apparent but his original inclination to move sideways and forward, to spread and advance, is now counterbalanced by frequent enclosing in gestures and retreating in postures. An increase in boundness and a tendency to shrink, a relative dearth of direct efforts, and a decrease of horizontal shaping have brought about a restriction in Charlie's attention, imagination, and exploration, especially in activities such as school work, for which he lacks motivation.

In his postural movements one can see even better than in gestures how much Charlie has become involved in defensive functioning. In postural movements his tension-flow becomes much more free than bound; the ratio of growing to shrinking augments to 4:1 whereas in gestures it is 1:2. Indirectness of effort and spreading in space increases twofold and enclosing ceases altogether. His native inclinations come through in these patterns; he uses them to wander off into a world of fantasy, unable to focus on what is in front of him. His fantasies seem to be primarily of an aggressive nature. His lightness decreases and he uses a great deal of strength combined with downward shaping and descending. Not only does he accelerate more in postures than in gestures, but deceleration, his long favored effort element, ceases altogether. At the same time his advancing decreases and retreat occurs five times as often as in gestures. These well-matched effort-shape combinations serve him well in his fights with his mother and teachers; whenever he can he runs away from obstacles instead of overcoming them but, when cornered, he stands his ground with stubborn determination. He appears to cope with the increase in his drives by resisting or avoiding the challenges of reality and retreating into a world of fantasy.

Charlie's native abilities, his superior capacity to integrate, and his total involvement in what he is doing (29, 30) are expressed in the richness of his effort-shape repertoire, in the balance between related effort and shaping elements, and in his superior performance in postural movements. The high degree of affinity between qualities of tension-flow and shape-flow, efforts and shaping indicates that the level of Charlie's object-relationships is well integrated with the quality of his ego attitudes. The consistent use of well-matched motion factors in postures reflects Charlie's ego strength in states of high motivation. The discrepancy between his performance in postures and gestures outlines a large area of conflicts which cause Charlie to spend much of his energy in maintaining a highly cathected defense organization.[9]

---

[9] Assessment of Charlie's rhythms of tension-flow suggests that a recent influx of oral sadism threatens his phallic position which is already weakened by a predominantly oro-anal drive organization. Newly acquired insight about differences between pure rhythms ('oral', 'anal', 'phallic', etc.) and mixed rhythms ('oro-anal', 'oro-phallic', etc.) allows a better retrospective evaluation of Charlie's drive development. I had interpreted Charlie's originally preferred rhythm of tension-flow as a variety of an 'anal' rhythm (29, 30); at this time I would classify it as a mixed 'oro-anal-sadistic' rhythm.

Possibly because of an inertia due to illness, noted during the last visit, Charlie's mother sits down more frequently than before; she seems subdued and she hardly uses efforts and shaping in postures. Directness, lightness, and acceleration give her movements a quality of dabbing, but none of these efforts is matched in quantity by appropriate shaping. She still tends to move upward or retreat but there is too little shape-flow and shaping for the amount of tension and effort she generates. This suggests a deficiency in adaptation to objects.

Charlie is now taller than his mother and likes to talk to her standing up and looking down at her. When she criticizes him, he puts her in her place and she yields. But there is better attunement between them since Charlie uses as many changes in tension-flow as she does. His increased acceleration accommodates his mother's preferred effort so that their timing is well coördinated. She responds to him with pleasure, looking up to him as they still 'vibrate' together in an intense affective interchange initiated by Charlie. Their roles seem to be reversed as he towers over her, subdues her, and retreats from her even more often than she does from him. Much of his present behavior repeats the domination of his mother when he was a toddler.

Glenda's interaction with her mother falls within the range of normalcy; Nancy's behavior is deviant but not easy to label; Charlie's neurotic development was already evident in his first year of life. In all three diagnostic categories it is possible to use movement profiles for the assessment of personality traits.

SUMMARY

The study of shapes of the body and their changes in rhythms of shape-flow contributes to our understanding of feeling tones that emerge from kinesthetic sensations in infancy. Growing and shrinking of body shape serve approach and withdrawal behavior. Regulation of shape-flow through physiological and psychological mechanisms contributes to the formation of images of self and object. In the state of primary narcissism the prevailing tendency is toward shrinking of body shape or turning inward. As development progresses there is an increasing tendency toward growing of body shape and thus turning to the environment.

In the near body space in which mother and infant interact, the affective milieu is created by mutual attunement in rhythms of tension-flow and by reciprocal adjustment of rhythms of shape-flow. The infant turns to the source of satisfaction but his reaching for the need-satisfying object is not yet intentionally directed. As 'directional' and intentional movements become possible through maturation of apparatus and repeated experiences of distance from the mother, the child localizes the object in space; he recognizes its sameness in the 'near space', the 'reach space', and the 'general space' as well. When ambivalence to the object prevails, the child's ability to weigh, appraise, and discriminate can maintain object constancy despite contradictory qualities of the object and changing feeling tones. When locomotion allows the child to explore the general space, a newly acquired sense of continuity in time and space increases his self-confidence and establishes a continuity of relationship despite the mobility of self and object.

In the oral phase, communication between mother and child is initiated and terminated through transactions in the horizontal, the feeding plane which remains the preferred plane of communication throughout life. In the anal stage, the stability of images of self and object is enhanced by mastery of gravity and transactions in the vertical plane in which children and adults present their true intent. In the urethral phase, timely decisions are best made through progression or retreat in the sagittal plane which is the plane of choice for operational transactions.

In an early 'inner-genital' phase, pregenital trends become integrated with genital impulses and inner genital sensations are externalized. At that time fantasies about the 'inside' of the body are structured by play configurations that help to establish spatial relations. In the phallic phase the child intrudes into space with his whole body; he identifies outside space with his love object.

In latency, the increasing harmony in the ego expresses itself in progressive integration of motions. 'Efforts' that reflect attitudes to space, gravity, and time, regulate the flow of tension; and shaping, in spatial directions and planes, regulates the flow of shape. The child coördinates these patterns of movement in the same measure as he solidifies conflict-free relations to objects through aim-inhibited drive discharge. In adolescence a chaotic disorganization of movement patterns is counteracted by maturation of apparatus that allow the expression of independent attitudes in postural movements.

In adulthood when genital dominance is reached, ego traits become permanent and relations to objects attain the highest degree of constancy. A harmonious integration of movement patterns in gestures and postures reflects the relatively conflict-free interaction between self and objects.

The repertoire of movement patterns can be represented in profiles that reveal the ratio between various motion factors used by an individual. Preferences for certain combinations and sequences of movement elements mark the individuality of drive constellations, of adaptation to the environment, and of adjustment to objects. Differences in styles of movement are determined by congenital preferences and kinesthetic identifications with love objects that evolve in progressive developmental stages.

Vignettes taken from movement profiles of three mothers and their children illustrate the way interaction through movement can reveal normal, deviant, and neurotic development.

REFERENCES

1. BALINT, ALICE: *Über eine besondere Form der infantilen Angst.* Ztschr. Psa. Paid., VII, 1933, pp. 414-417.
2. BALINT, MICHAEL: *Thrills and Regressions.* New York: International Universities Press, Inc., 1959.
3. ———: *Primary Narcissism and Primary Love.* This QUARTERLY, XXIX, 1960, pp. 6-43.

4. BARTENIEFF, IRMA and DAVIS, MARTHA: *Effort-Shape Analysis of Movement.* Unpublished.

5. BENEDEK, THERESE: *Adaptation to Reality in Early Infancy.* This QUARTERLY, VII, 1938, pp. 200-214.

6. BIRDWHISTELL, RAY L.: *Kinesics Analysis in the Investigation of Emotion.* Amer. Assn. Advancement of Science, 1960.

7. BRIERLEY, MARJORIE: *Trends in Psychoanalysis.* London: Hogarth Press, 1951.

8. BUEHLER, KARL: *The Mental Development of the Child.* New York: Harcourt, Brace & Co., 1930.

9. BURLINGHAM, DOROTHY: *Psychoanalytische Beobachtungen an blinden Kindern.* Int. Ztschr. f. Psa., XXV, 1940, pp. 297-335.

10. CALL, JUSTIN: *Newborn Approach Behavior and Early Ego Development.* Int. J. Psa., XLV, 1964, pp. 286-293.

11. DARWIN, CHARLES: *The Expression of the Emotions in Man and Animals.* New York: Philosophical Library, Inc., 1955.

12. DEUTSCH, FELIX: *Analysis of Postural Behavior.* This QUARTERLY, XVI, 1947, pp. 195-213.

13. ———: *Thus Speaks the Body. I. An Analysis of Postural Behavior.* Trans. New York Acad. Science, Series 2, XII, 1950.

14. ———: *Thus Speaks the Body. III. Analytic Posturology.* Presented at meeting of the New York Psa. Society. Abstracted in This QUARTERLY, XX, 1951, pp. 338-339.

15. ERIKSON, ERIK H.: *Sex Differences in the Play Configurations of a Representative Group of Preadolescents.* Amer. J. Orthopsychiatry, XXI, 1951, pp. 667-692.

16. ———: *Identity and the Life Cycle.* Psychological Issues, I. New York: International Universities Press, Inc., 1959.

17. FREUD, ANNA: The Mutual Influences in the Development of Ego and Id. In: *The Psychoanalytic Study of the Child, Vol. VII.* New York: International Universities Press, Inc., 1952, pp. 43-50.

18. ———: *Normality and Pathology in Childhood.* New York: International Universities Press, Inc., 1965.

19. FREUD: *On Narcissism* (1914). Standard Edition, XIV.

20. ———: *Instincts and Their Vicissitudes* (1915). Standard Edition, XIV.

21. ———: *Introductory Lectures on Psychoanalysis* (1917). Standard Edition, XV and XVI.

22. ———: *Beyond the Pleasure Principle* (1920). Standard Edition, XVIII.

23. HARTMANN, HEINZ: The Mutual Influences in the Development of the Ego and the Id. In: *The Psychoanalytic Study of the Child, Vol. VII.* New York: International Universities Press, Inc., 1952, pp. 7-30.

24. HERMANN, IMRE: *Sich-Anklammern, Auf-Suche Gehen.* Ztschr. f. Psa., XXII, 1936, pp. 349-370.

25. HOFFER, WILLI: The Mutual Influences in the Development of the Ego and the Id. In: *The Psychoanalytic Study of the Child, Vol. VII.* New York: International Universities Press, Inc., 1952, pp. 31-42.

26. JACOBSON, EDITH: *The Self and the Object World*. New York: International Universities Press, Inc., 1964.

27. JOFFE, W. G. and SANDLER, JOSEPH: *Disorders of Narcissism*. Read at the Mid-winter Meeting of the Amer. Psa. Assn., 1965.

28. KESTENBERG, JUDITH S.: *History of an 'Autistic Child'*. J. Child Psychiatry, II, 1953, pp. 5-52.

29. ———: *The Role of Movement Patterns in Development. I. Rhythms of Movement*. This QUARTERLY, XXXIV, 1965, pp. 1-36.

30. ———: *The Role of Movement Patterns in Development. II. Flow of Tension and Effort*. This QUARTERLY, XXXIV, 1965, pp. 517-563.

31. ———: *Rhythm and Organization in Obsessive-Compulsive Development*. Read at the Meeting of the International Psychoanalytic Congress, 1965.

32. ———: *Movement Profiles*. In preparation.

33. KRIS, ERNST: *Ein geisteskranker Bildhauer*. Imago, XIX, 1933, pp. 384-411.

34. LABAN, RUDOLF: *Modern Educational Dance*. London: MacDonald & Evans, 1948.

35. ———: *The Mastery of Movement*. Second edition. Revised and enlarged by Lisa Ullman. London: MacDonald & Evans, 1960.

36. LAMB, WARREN: *Posture and Gesture*. London: Gerald Duckworth & Co. Ltd., 1965.

37. LEWIN, BERTRAM D.: *The Psychoanalysis of Elation*. New York: The Psychoanalytic Quarterly, Inc., 1961.

38. LICHTENSTEIN, HEINZ: *The Role of Narcissism in the Emergence and Maintenance of Primary Identity*. Int. J. Psa., XLV, 1964, pp. 49-56.

39. MAHLER, MARGARET S.: On Child Psychosis and Schizophrenia. In: *The Psychoanalytic Study of the Child, Vol. VII*. New York: International Universities Press, Inc., 1952, pp. 252-261.

40. ———: Thoughts about Development and Individuation. In: *The Psychoanalytic Study of the Child, Vol. XVIII*. New York: International Universities Press, Inc., 1963, pp. 307-324.

41. NORTH, MARIAN: *A Simple Guide to Movement Teaching*. London: Marian North, 1959.

42. PRECHTL, H. F. R.: *Die Entwicklung und Eigenart fruehkindlicher Bewegungsweisen*. Klinische Wochenschrft., XXXIV, 1956, pp. 281-284.

43. ——— and SCHLEIDT, W. M.: *Ausloesende und Steuernde Mechanismen des Saugaktes*. Ztschr. f. Vergleichende Physiologie, XXXII, 1950, pp. 257-262; XXXIII, 1951, pp. 53-62.

44. PRESTON, VALERIE: *A Handbook for Modern Educational Dance*. London: MacDonald & Evans, 1963.

45. RUSSEL, JOAN: *Modern Dance in Education*. London: MacDonald & Evans, 1958.

46. SANDLER, JOSEPH and ROSENBLATT, B.: The Concept of the Representational World. In: *The Psychoanalytic Study of the Child, Vol. XVII*. New York: International Universities Press, Inc., 1962, pp. 287-291.

47. SCHILDER, PAUL: *Image and Appearance of the Human Body*. Psyche Monographs No. 4. London: Kegan Paul, Trench, Trubner & Co., 1935.

48. SCHNEIRLA, T. C.: An Evolutionary and Developmental Theory of Biphasic Processes Underlying Approach and Withdrawal. In: *Nebraska Symposium on Motivation*. Lincoln: University of Nebraska Press, 1959, pp. 1-42.

49. SHERRINGTON, C. S.: *The Integrative Action of the Nervous System*. New Haven: Yale University Press, 1923.

50. SPIEGEL, LEO: The Self, the Sense of Self, and Perception. In: *The Psychoanalytic Study of the Child, Vol. XIV*. New York: International Universities Press, Inc., 1959, pp. 81-109.

51. SPITZ, RENÉ: *No and Yes*. New York: International Universities Press, Inc., 1957.

52. ———: in collaboration with Cobliner, Godfrey: *The First Year of Life*. New York: International Universities Press, Inc., 1965.

53. WOLFF, PETER H. and WHITE, BURTON L.: *Visual Pursuit and Attention in Young Infants*. J. Acad. Child Psychiatry, IV, 1965, pp. 473-485.

The Role of Movement Patterns in Development
in Development
Vol. 2

EPILOGUE AND GLOSSARY

by
Judith S. Kestenberg, M.D.

Clinical Professor of Psychiatry
Downstate Medical Center, Brooklyn, N.Y.

Pediatric Psychiatrist
Long Island Jewish-Hillside Medical Center, New Hyde Park, N.Y.

Co-Director
Center for Parents and Children, Roslyn, N.Y.
Operated by Child Development Research, Sands Point, N.Y.*

with the collaboration of
K. Mark Sossin

Doctoral Candidate in Clinical Psychology
Yeshiva University, New York, N.Y.

*Royalties from the sale of this book will help support Research, Service and Training Programs at the Center for Parents and Children.

NEW YORK 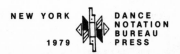 DANCE
NOTATION
BUREAU
1979 PRESS

Copyright © 1979
by
Judith S. Kestenberg and K. Mark Sossin
All rights reserved

Library of Congress Catalog Card Number: 78-67319
ISBN 0-932582-01-X

Printed in the United States of America

Dance Notation Bureau, Inc.
505 Eighth Avenue
New York, New York 10018

TABLE OF CONTENTS

LIST OF ILLUSTRATIONS

INTRODUCTION

A longitudinal study of three children, described in the first volume (Kestenberg, 1965-67), was begun with the express purpose of devising a system of notation and categorization of movement patterns which would be applicable to babies, children and adults. Through the twenty years of this study, we learned to discriminate between various patterns and developed methods of notating them in isolation from one another. Even though the mothers had many mature patterns which their infants had not yet acquired, one could compare parents and infants by singling out those patterns they both had at their disposal. With progressive maturation, children tended to use some of their newly acquired patterns more often than others. However, the degree to which this occurred varied not only in accordance with their own predispositions, but also in accordance with their mothers' preferences.

In this epilogue, I shall compare the data I obtained during these children's infancy with those I observed during their latency, early adolescence and near adulthood. Early assessments were based on crude recordings of movement and on clinical impressions. Assessments made in late latency, in early adolescence and later were based on comparable movement profiles (MP).

I shall try to list the advancements in movement notation and interpretation which have been made since the first attempts to notate and describe the interaction between the infantile and maternal preferences for certain rhythms. To give structure to the vast array of old and new data, I shall arrange chapters in accordance with questions posed at the end of the first ten years of this study (Kestenberg, 1965, p. 34):

1. Preferences for Certain Rhythms of Movement in Early Infancy.

2. Maturational and Environmental Influences that Modify the Originally Preferred Rhythms.

3. Early Manifestations of Disturbed Development Due to Clashes Between the Rhythms of Infant and Mother.

4. Later Behavior which can be Derived from Motor Rhythms.

1

5. Identification of Specific Motor Rhythms as Expressive of Specific Drives such as Oral, Anal, Phallic and Others.

6. Transitions Between Drive and Ego Dependent Motility.

7. Methods of Notation that would Permit Objective Differentiation Between Rhythmic Discharge of Tension and the More Mature Components of Movement which serve Complex Ego Functions.

Some of the chapters will be short and others quite long, some familiar and others new, but in all the reader will become reacquainted with the three children of this study. The last reports (vol. I. 1967, pp. 128-133) on Glenda, Nancy and Charlie were dated in their early adolescence. The last profiles on which this epilogue is based were constructed when they were nearly twenty years old. Clinical vignettes of these young people when they were entering the life of adulthood will serve as an introduction to the epilogue.

Glenda, Charlie and Nancy at the End of

Their Adolescence.

As her adolescence progressed, Glenda increasingly came to resemble her mother. From an abrupt, stringbean-type of girl, she developed into a soft, wider, curvaceous and feminine looking young lady. Her smile was charming and a happy expression predominated even when she was a bit anxious. Her abruptness was noticeable when she suddenly came up with a new idea or linked what she had just said to a new thought.

When she was over eighteen, Glenda became engaged, and a few months after the engagement she was married. When I saw her just before her twentieth birthday she was at the end of the middle trimester of pregnancy. Although she had become independent before marriage, pregnancy brought her closer to her mother, who resumed scolding and taunting her. Her mother's remark, that Glenda started things without finishing them, reminded me of early maternal complaints about baby-Glenda who fell asleep without finishing her bottle. Glenda protested, but made it apparent that she still worked in phases of great involvement which were then followed by rest or change of occupation. This innate biphasic rhythmicity seemed unrelated to the task at hand. Glenda was anxious but had spurts of cheerfulness in anticipation of her baby.

Charlie, at the age of almost twenty, has grown into a tall, broad shouldered adolescent with narrow hips. In the last phase of adolescence, as he approached adulthood, Charlie's body contours have become more defined. At the same time, he has become independent of his parents and has found gainful employment. For the time being, he has simply withdrawn from further formal learning, as he did in his infancy when the overstimulation of a noisy kitchen proved to be more than he could handle. However, his talent for organizing and absorbing a great deal, when met on his terms, has remained as a permanent character trait. During the interview, he spoke very little but did become animated in a conversation about his girl-friend and his sister. Generally quiet and deliberate-looking, he moved abruptly when he was stimulated, when he teased, or when he told a joke. Moving gradually and slowly, he observed what was going on around him, even though he sometimes gave the impression that he was not listening.

With increasing maturity, Nancy, at the age of almost twenty, lost much of her original rigidity. She not only finished high-school with great success, but also enrolled in college. In late adolescence, Nancy had overcome her reticence and had learned partially to control the incessant fiddling of her hands and feet. Most characteristic of her demeanor in the last interview was her shyness with strangers and her animation with her sisters and numerous brothers. If a topic was of great interest to her, Nancy was able to use a variety of advanced movement patterns, involving a high degree of complexity. However, these occasions were rare and difficult to predict. For example, Nancy turned to me unexpectedly and asked about the nature of my project. Sometimes, she pursued this interest with long questions and appropriate gesticulations, but at other times she spoke about it in monosyllables only and became immobile, as she did in her childhood. Her development appeared impressive as were her letters, written with skill and a good vocabulary. What used to be perseveration expresses itself now in repetitiousness and in a difficulty in the preparation of new phrases and transitions between phrases. What had been described as rigidity could still be identified as such in the way Nancy keeps her trunk still when she gesticulates with her limbs.

CHAPTER 1

PREFERENCES FOR CERTAIN RHYTHMS OF
MOVEMENT IN EARLY INFANCY

A rhythm, in whatever motor or sensory form it appears, is a temporal pattern in which individual units, repeated periodically, are more or less consistently varied in any one or more of their qualitative and quantitative attributes (Ruckmick, 1923). Motor rhythms, as described here, do not pertain to periods of movement alternating with rest but rather to alternations of simple qualities of tension or repetitions of complex sequential and quantitatively differing units of tension. Simple alternations of free and bound flow are characteristic of sinus rhythms which are suitable for oral-type discharge forms such as sucking. Notating "oral" rhythms, we find that their simplest units are representable as arcs in free flow ⌒ or in bound flow ⌣. When repeated, these units form sequences such as these: ⌒⌣⌒⌣. An example of a complex rhythmic unit is seen in the notation of straining rhythms which are suitable for anal-sadistic-type discharge forms. Notating this type of rhythm, we find that the duration of its units is longer than that of "oral" rhythms. In addition, they display greater variability. They all have in common the holding of a given intensity of tension on an even level, for some time: ⎯⎯⌣⎯⎯ or ⎯⎯⌣ or ⎯⌒⎯ The variable factors are: the intensity, which is usually high but occasionally low; the steepness or graduality of ascent; and the sequence of changes from free to bound flow and vice versa. These rhythms can follow each other, as for instance, in repeated straining during defecation. The interval between repetitions is varied, from a few seconds to hours. A "phallic" rhythmic unit is characterized by the abruptness of ascent and descent of tension. When notated during masturbation or during jumping it consists of oscillating units following each other in quick succession:

. However, it can occur as a single unit which may not be repeated for some time, as, for example in:

Preferences

At the beginning of this study, the data obtained were crude and could be detected without reliable notation. However, there was no doubt that each of the three infants preferred his own type of rhythmicity. Since that time, we have learned to notate much more accurately and are able to obtain comparable results from different notators.

By computing the rhythmic units contained in a representative sample of tension-flow notations, one can obtain ratios between them, for instance oral:anal: phallic = 4:1:2 or 3:2:1. One can thus see whether there is an even distribution of rhythms or whether there is a preference for one or more rhythmic units which are repeated more often than others. As a result, one can obtain data that can be used to assess preferential constellations of motor discharge forms rather than just simple preferences.

Our present method of quantifying and diagramming rhythms of tension-flow is a considerable advancement over the first crude attempts to classify rhythms as "oral", "anal" or "phallic". In addition, we have been able to detect many more types of rhythms than was possible in the beginning of the study. As our observations progressed, we could distinguish between rhythms serving libidinal needs and those serving sadistic needs. Although we could usefully apply Laban's (1947) polarity between "fighting" and "indulging" effort elements and subdivide tension-flow attributes similarly, we could not do the same for the division of rhythms. None of us[1] could identify rhythmic units which were suitable for the expression of unadulterated aggression. We have come to the conclusion that purely aggressive rhythmic discharge forms do not exist or cannot be noted with our present methods of observation. Therefore, we have followed the classification of subphases as "libidinal" (that is, predominantly libidinal) and "sadistic" (Freud, 1917; Abraham, 1924), and we have named the rhythmic units after the phases and zones in which they predominate in all children. In doing so, we discovered that each "libidinal" rhythm had its counterpart in a "sadistic" rhythm. We also discovered through movement notation, clinical observations and psychoanalyses (Kestenberg, 1969) that there is an orderly sequence of subphases in which periods of predominantly "libidinal" rhythms preceed periods of predominantly "sadistic" rhythms in each developmental phase.

---

[1] In the Sands Point Movement Study Group: Dr. J. Berlowe Mrs. A. Buelte, Dr. J. Kestenberg, Dr. H. Marcus and Dr. E. Robbins.

In the first year of life we saw that the predominance of "oral" sucking rhythms

waned as the "oral-sadistic" snapping and **biting** rhythms

increased.

"Anal" twisting rhythms

which prevailed at the end of the first year and the beginning of the second, became less frequent when "anal-sadistic" straining rhythms

were more prominent in the latter part of the second year. Surprisingly, the same was true of "phallic" rhythms.

Jumping-type phallic rhythms

the clarity and frequency of which came to a peak between the ages of four and five, became relatively less frequent a year later when leaping-type "phallic-sadistic" rhythms

were more intense and more frequent

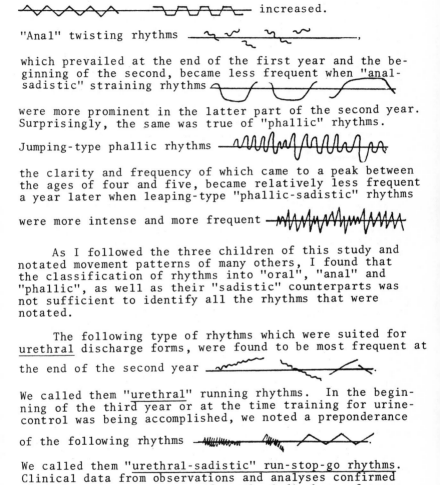

As I followed the three children of this study and notated movement patterns of many others, I found that the classification of rhythms into "oral", "anal" and "phallic", as well as their "sadistic" counterparts was not sufficient to identify all the rhythms that were notated.

The following type of rhythms which were suited for urethral discharge forms, were found to be most frequent at

the end of the second year

We called them "urethral" running rhythms. In the beginning of the third year or at the time training for urine-control was being accomplished, we noted a preponderance

of the following rhythms

We called them "urethral-sadistic" run-stop-go rhythms. Clinical data from observations and analyses confirmed that there were two types of urethral discharge forms: 1) The pleasurable letting-yourself-go, during absence or loss of sphincter control; and 2) The pleasurable controlled shooting of urine with the intent to injure.

7

The following rhythms were first discovered in little girls between the ages of two-and-a-half and four: . They were seen more frequently in women than in men and we called them feminine undulating rhythms. Subsequently, Robbins and Soodak (personal communication) discovered the same rhythms in the tunica Dartos of the scrotum. We renamed them "inner-genital" feminine undulating rhythms[2] in accordance with our clinical finding that an inner-genital phase precedes the phallic in both sexes (the girl's lasting longer than that of the boy). The much more intense inner-genital swaying rhythm

is similar to uterine contractions and releases. It is seen more often at the end of the inner-genital phase, but we never found it to be more frequent than other rhythms except during labor and delivery. We can refer to it as "inner-genital-sadistic" in accordance with its ex-pulsive quality and in correlation with the sadistic fantasies of parturients (Kestenberg, 1976), which give rise to fears that the child or the mother's genital will be mutilated.

The prototypes for "oral" and "oral-sadistic" rhythms are "sucking" and "biting" respectively. The prototypes for "anal" and "anal-sadistic" rhythms are an "anal-sphincter" type of "twisting" and "straining" respectively. The prototypes for "urethral" and "urethral-sadistic" rhythms are "running" and "run-stop-run" rhythms. The prototypes for "inner-genital-libidinal" and "inner-genital-sadistic" rhythms are "undulating" and "swaying" (feminine-type rhythms). The prototypes for "phallic" and "phallic-sadistic" type rhythms are "jumping" and "leaping".

On the basis of these and similar studies, it is possible to say that there is a relationship between preferences for certain rhythms and certain types of organization. The use of many short-lived rhythmic units ("oral" or "phallic") connotes a tendency towards simple repetitiousness or rapid synthesis. In sequences of such rhythms and rest, we detect tendencies towards a bi-phasic organization. A preference for rhythmic units of long duration ("anal-sadistic" and "inner-

---

[2] Before this discovery, we tended to classify these rhythms as "anal" or "anal-sadistic" and later as mixed "oral-anal". This error was especially signi-ficant in Charlie's case.

genital") suggests an aptitude for retention or integration[3].

Nancy's preference for "oral-sadistic" rhythms was linked with her tendency to perseverate and condense. Both are still in evidence.

Glenda's preference for "phallic" rhythms, followed by rest periods or by short bouts of "oral-sadistic" rhythms, initiated her bi-phasic organization which still persists.

Charlie's preference for "inner-genital" rhythms seems to have contributed to his ability to centralize and integrate, which is still in evidence.

Section I

Pure, Mixed and Modified Rhythms

We call rhythms, described above, pure because of their close correspondence to their prototypes. In contrast, we call rhythms in which one can detect the confluence or combination of various pure rhythms mixed rhythms. An example of confluence is an "oro-phallic" rhythmic unit which displays both the arc of the oral rhythm $(\frown o)$ and the abruptness of the phallic $(\sqcap p)$. However, the oral arc has changed its character by the influence of abruptness, and the intensity of the phallic rhythm is muted, resulting in $\frown$ op op . An example of

three rhythms combining with one another is an "anal-sadistic -- anal -- oral-sadistic" rhythm

in which the even level typical for a straining rhythm is

---

[3] It is not possible to expand here further on the connection between rhythms and organization. The reader is referred to a paper on this topic (Kestenberg, 1969) and to a chapter on adolescent rhythmicity in my book "Children and Parents" (Kestenberg & Robbins, 1975).

modified by the addition of sequences of "anal" and
"oral-sadistic" rhythms. All of the rhythmic units
which are added retain their pure form but are forced
into the course taken by the "anal-sadistic" rhythm
which organizes and limits them.

Originally, we used to distinguish between pure
and modified rhythms. The assumption was made that one
rhythm was altered by another to accommodate to a given
function or to alter it. We have learned since that
there are many ways in which rhythmic units combine,
and we are not certain of the purpose of such combinations. We can still speak of a modified rhythm when we
can clearly recognize the original form of a pure rhythmic unit which has been changed through attunement with
someone else's rhythm. A baby, using an "anal-sadistic"
rhythm may incorporate into it his mother's "oral-
sadistic" and "anal" components, as seen in the illustration above.

Section II

Mixed, Organizing and Derailed Rhythms

Analysts have long been aware that various drive
components can become condensed. A wish, expressed in
oral terms, may be a cover for a genital wish or vice
versa. The dominant wish betrays itself through the mode
of its organization. For instance, a fantasy of delaying ejaculation for a very long time, betrays its primary
derivation from an anal-sadistic drive component. Sometimes, the intermingling of two or three types of wishes
suggests that they are all of equal valence to the
patient. There are patients who habitually mix ideational content in such a way that their thoughts interrupt,
derail and disorganize each other. A parallel process
occurs in rhythmic motor discharge. Mixed rhythms - the
motor correlates of mixed drive components - result from
additions, condensations, combinations and confluences.

Long lasting rhythmic units have an organizing effect
upon other rhythmic components which they can incorporate
without changing their original course too much. Sometimes, two rhythmic units create compromise forms. For

instance a "phallic" ⋀ rhythm will combine with an

"inner-genital" ⌣ to produce a mixed "phallic-

inner-genital" rhythm 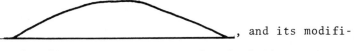. As discovered by
H. Marcus (personal communication), these mixed units
constitute the bulk of adult genital rhythms.   In
contrast to the smoothness with which these two rhythms
are synthesized to create a new unit, are malformed
derailed rhythms which cannot be fitted into any cate-
gory or seem to be mixtures of all rhythmic units 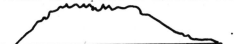 .

It is instructive to recall our successive interpretations of Charlie's preferred rhythms, as
reconstructed in the beginning of this study
(1965, vol. 1, p. 16). Reproduced here schematically is his unmodified preferred rhythmic unit:

, and its modifi-

cation in response to maternal stimulation:

.

In 1965 (p. 49), I said cautiously that Charlie's
preferred rhythm had certain features in common with
typical "anal" and "anal-sadistic" rhythms. At that
time it was thought that a gradual increase and decrease of tension was a characteristic of these
rhythms. Today, we classify very gradually rising
and falling wavy rhythms as "inner-genital". In the
modified rhythm above, we see a decrease in the
graduality of ascent and descent of tension and an
addition of numerous "oral", "oral-sadistic", "anal"
and "urethral" rhythmic units, which congregate on
a plateau, reminiscent of anal-sadistic rhythms.
If the curve, as drawn, is truly representative of
the effect of maternal stimulation on Charlie's
preferred rhythms, we would have to assume that a
modification has occurred as a result of strain
during the attunement with mother's abrupt "phallic"
and many other short-lived rhythmic units. We are
impressed with the integration of so many divergent rhythmic fluctuations which do not derail
Charlie's preferred rhythm and do not change its
course significantly.

Charlie's dialogue with his mother put him under considerable strain, but his vibrating excitement bore witness to
his capacity to relate in early infancy. Quite different were Nancy's "irregular staccato rhythms" which made
her behavior bizarre from the start.

Nancy could be described as a dysrhythmic baby. From the difficulty I had in reconstructing them, I suspect that many of her rhythms were derailed. In 1965 I referred to them as 'oral-sadistic', mixed with other unidentifiable rhythms" (p. 49). I depicted them in the following manner:

Today we would score some of these rhythms as "phallic", some as "anal-sadistic", mixed with "oral", "oral-sadistic", a few "anal", "urethral-sadistic" and "phallic-sadistic" components, following and derailing one another.

Pure and mixed rhythms are observable at birth and in fetal movement. There are many more derailed rhythms in immature, vulnerable and disorganized babies than in average infants. There is a progressive trend from the mixture of many types of rhythms, which may interrupt and derail one another, to harmonious combinations of only two rhythmic units. Another significant discovery is that, in the first day of life, one can frequently notice mixtures of two or more "sadistic" rhythmic units. On the second neonatal day, this trend already disappears and mixed rhythms begin to contain more "libidinal" than "sadistic" rhythm components. This is generally true in normal development. "Sadistic" components are more apt to predominate in pure rhythms. For instance, the ratio between pure "libidinal" and "sadistic" rhythms may be 1:2. The reverse is true of mixed rhythms. Their ratio may be 2:1. Except at the height of "sadistic" phases and in pathological conditions, "libidinal" rhythms predominate in mixed rhythms.

Our preliminary findings suggest that preferences for certain rhythms of movement can be detected early and can also be traced into adulthood where they appear frequently in mixed rhythms. Rhythms, encouraged by the mother or enhanced by current biological forces, appear frequently in pure rhythms. At times, babies show clear preferences for certain rhythms, be they pure or mixed, while at other times we can detect certain rhythm constellations which can be defined in terms of ratios, sequences and modifiability. We can, for instance, speak of an early predilection for phallic rhythms, as was seen in Glenda; we can study how a preferred rhythm changes under the influence of the mother, as was seen in Charlie; and we can detect a predisposition to sadistic discharge forms, as was seen in Nancy. We can investigate which rhythmic units tend to follow one another and we can describe the activities in which certain rhythms tend to be used.

CHAPTER 2

MATURATIONAL AND ENVIRONMENTAL INFLUENCES
THAT MODIFY THE ORIGINALLY PREFERRED RHYTHMS

All rhythms can be noted in the newborn and preferences for certain rhythms can be detected early. Through
the notation and scoring of movement patterns in different age groups, both in this country and in Israeli
Kibbutzim, I recognized that oral rhythms are most frequent in the oral phase, and usually remain the most
frequent throughout life. However, rhythm distribution
is affected by maturation. For instance, "anal" rhythms
are most frequent in the anal phase, the "urethral"
rhythms in the urethral phase, and so on.

During the neonatal phase, "oral" rhythms become better differentiated and, in the oral phase, they predominate in their pure form. Sucking in an "oral" rhythm
and biting in an "oral-sadistic" rhythm are biologically
advantageous. However, there are many other activities
for which "oral" rhythms are quite suitable. The whole
snout-region makes use of them. For instance, perioral
muscles contract and relax in an "oral" rhythm during
speech. When "oral-sadistic" or "anal-sadistic" rhythms
invade and interfere with the "oral", speech can become
"biting" or "strained". "Urethral" rhythms help to slur
speech; "inner-genital" introduce a drawl and "phallic"
make speech explosive. We note these influences in successive developmental phases.

Orality, which is the first organization of the
child, remains dominant even after new phases and advanced
patterns have been introduced through maturation and
learning. This dominance can be partially accounted for
by the fact that oral rhythms tend to repeat themselves
and are used in repetitive activities, especially in the
peripheral regions of the body, such as face, fingers
and toes. Before one can postulate an oral fixation or
regression one must be sufficiently experienced to know
by how much oral rhythms usually exceed others.

When the original preferences are so strong that
they overshadow the maturational influx of phase-specific
rhythms, development is marred by early fixation.

When the influence of maturation is of greater importance than the fixation, as for instance during pregnancy, the originally preferred rhythms decrease in
proportion to those prevalent at this time (see Glenda's

13

profile, p.129). An example of a deviant record, in which mixed rhythms are very scanty, can be seen in Nancy's profile (p.131).

The influence of maternal rhythmic patterns is another means by which the original ratio of rhythms is modified. Through attunement with his mother, the baby begins to move increasingly in rhythms his mother likes. Since all of them exist in his repertoire from the beginning, he is capable of reproducing those to which he is exposed frequently. There is something contagious about rhythmic repetition, especially when there is an intimate contact between two bodies. With the help of his mother, the infant learns to apply rhythms in an optimal "pure" way, at a time, when and, in a zone, where they are biologically most advantageous. Thus the sucking rhythm called for during nursing becomes synchronized with the frequency of maternal milk-expulsion. At the same time, maternal and infantile movements display an oral rhythm in rocking, fingering, tapping and breathing. Maternal rhythms have the greatest impact upon the infant when they operate in specific zones, in conjunction with specific activities. This leads to a phase-specific differentiation of rhythms.

Because mothers care for all their babies' needs from the start, they prime them, for the use of specific rhythms in specific zones, before maturation promotes their differentiation. Wiping the babies' anus, mothers use anal rhythms; they may deliberately strain to help a baby defecate before they begin toilet training. When mothers prematurely or belatedly "push" phase-inappropriate rhythms, they encourage a fixation or regression in the child. Because maternal teaching is an aid to differentiation, rhythms favored by the mother are frequently dominant in pure rhythms.

Contact with the mother's "libidinal" rhythms promotes a rapid desaggressivization of mixed rhythmic discharge-forms after birth. The newborn is still flooded with placental hormones and his tension-flow rhythms are influenced by them. In the first few days of life and often longer, "inner-genital" rhythms predominate over others, with the exception of the oral. This guarantees a certain similarity between maternal and infantile rhythms which makes the baby familiar to the mother and vice versa. By the time the sex hormones are excreted and the "inner-genital" rhythms become considerably reduced, the baby's oral rhythms are usually well differentiated.

All that has been said about rhythms so far pertained to tension-flow rhythms. In surveying other rhythms, we note that there is a progressive tendency to

use more centrifugal than centripetal movements. An inborn attraction between hand and mouth, and between
thighs and pelvis is at first counteracted by a lack of
control over shape-flow and tension-flow. Once they
reach the mouth, hands are derailed in the opposite direction; legs flex and extend in an irregular fashion.
There is little coordination between upper and lower
rhythms until the baby learns to keep his finger in his
mouth. Staring in corners and watching hands stabilizes
the baby, reducing flow fluctuations both in tension-
and in shape-flow. A similar stabilizing effect is
derived from listening. Children who evidence a good
attention-span early in life and are easily calmed by
persistent visual or acoustic stimuli, have an innate
capacity to keep tension on an even level or to re-
adjust it in a fine way. At the same time, they seem
to have a propensity for moving in the horizontal plane
by widening and narrowing. Most attentive seem to be
those whose favored rhythmic units are of long duration.
They either use even flow persistently or tend to be
very gradual. At the same time, inhalation and exhalation are prolonged, and turning to or away from stimuli
leads to certain body-shapes and positions, which are
maintained for some time. It seems that once these
babies react to a stimulus, they quickly become imper-
vious to the next one. Children, born with a great many
flow fluctuations are less attentive than their counterparts. They not only perpetually change their tension
quality, but also their shape and position. They frown,
pucker their lips, twist their nostrils, and raise their
eye-brows in quick succession, even when their limbs are
not in perpetual motion. The attentive infant roughly
corresponds to what Fries & Wolf (1958) call the "quiet
child", and the inattentive child corresponds to what
they call the "active child". The attentive child becomes more and more attentive with maturation until he
reaches the phallic phase when he becomes beset by conflicts between his innate and his phase-specific drive-
components. The restless, inattentive child profits
from maturation, which tends to decrease frequencies of
changes. These general trends become somewhat obscured
when one takes into account the many variables that influence individual development.

    Glenda's original preference for phallic rhythms
and her early ability to get into reach-space by
flinging her legs has undergone many changes throughout her development. I shall single out only those
for which I can account. Under the combined influence of her mother's rhythms and progressive
maturation, Glenda lost some of her phallic
abruptness. This was reinforced by her mother's
encouragement of stabilization at the time
Glenda began to stare at bright colors for a

long time. During her early phallic phase, Glenda
reacted to her brother's birth with an influx of
oral-sadistic impulses. This regression had the
prehistory of Glenda's early filling of her rest-
periods with fiddling, "oral-sadistic" rhythms.
Now she could get no rest, but was continuously on
the go. Whereas before, Glenda was abrupt but her
reversals from free to bound flow were smooth, now
she became angular, and soon she became beset by
an abundance of sharp phallic-sadistic rhythms.
Before her phallic phase, Glenda had played a great
deal with dolls and was very maternal. Retrospectively, I can recognize that she had many
inner-genital rhythms which served her maternality
well, but only one such instance was noted in the
record. However, at the time, these rhythms were
not classified yet and there were no profiles available to substantiate this impression. Similarly,
the influx of urethral rhythms, which made Glenda's
speech indistinct, was not acknowledged at the time.
Another source of modification of rhythms was the
maturation of efforts through which tension-flow
could be controlled as well as maturation of shaping
which controlled shape-flow rhythms. Especially in
latency, Glenda learned to subdue her natural tendencies in order to sit and do the disliked homework.
But not until she developed a greater facility in
the use of all effort elements in combinations, did
the contrast between her attitudes in play and work
become less marked.

Almost throughout her entire development, did
Glenda retain her proclivity for lengthening and
narrowing. The latter became less pronounced as a
narrow shape became part of Glenda's permanent body-
attitude. Maturation during adolescence brought
about Glenda's feminization whereby she seemed more
gradual and wider in her hips. Falling in love
further reinforced this trend. During her pregnancy,
Glenda widened a bit in the periphery, and despite
the fact that she sank in the middle (shortened)
like her mother, her tendency to lengthen persisted.
A year earlier, her pure rhythms betrayed a pregenital regression and an increase in "inner-genital"
rhythms at the expense of "phallic", but the mixed-
rhythm-ratio still showed a slight preference for the
latter. In the middle of her pregnancy, a regression to anality became most prominent, as evidenced
in her pure rhythms. However, the mixed-rhythm-
ratio revealed a decided preference for "inner-
genital" and "phallic" rhythms (see p.131).   The
maturational changes in pregnancy can account for
the changes in Glenda's recent rhythm repertoire

(Kestenberg, 1976), but the pre-pregnancy pregenital regression is more reminiscent of regressions,
initiating adulthood (Kestenberg, 1975).

Charlie's calm face, his broad shape and his
placid temperament did not change very much, except
during his growth spurt in adolescence. As a newborn he became entranced with hammering noises, and
he remained very quiet after his circumcision.
Much of his placidity was due to the frequency with
which he lapsed into neutral flow. He protected
himself against overstimulation by getting into
dazes, the prototypes of his later withdrawals. His
ability to attune to his mother's "phallic" rhythms
was instrumental in reducing his graduality. This
helped him to produce a mixed rhythmic unit which
resembled an "anal-sadistic" pattern, but still betrayed its derivation from an "inner-genital-sadistic"
pure rhythm. Into its plateau-like form he could
include many short-lived rhythmic units, among which
the oral were probably the most prominent. This
capacity came him in good stead in the oral phase
when most of his nourishment depended on bottle
feeding. During his inner-genital-phase, he seemed
saturated by "inner-genital" rhythms and he seemed to
have more "inner-genital-sadistic" rhythms at his
disposal than children generally have. At this time,
his maternality was reinforced by his identification
with his sister with whose dolls he played. Charlie
became more vivacious in the phallic phase and in the
beginning of adolescence. His latency was beset by
conflicts and prepuberty began with an oral-sadistic
regression which is still in evidence. The persistence of his preference for inner-genital rhythms
and their reduction in intensity staves off the dis-
ruptive influence of his (oral-sadistic) type of
restlessness which makes his fingers move beyond his
control. (See the many combinations of "sadistic"
rhythms with "inner-genital" in Charlie's profile
on p.130). Despite maturational changes and the
influence of his mother's and siblings' divergent
rhythms, Charlie has remained essentially the same
person, as far as his temperament is concerned. Perhaps, the influence of his calm and withdrawn father
has not been sufficiently taken into account in this
respect.

Maturation and growth had brought many changes
to Charlie's shape-flow and body-attitude. (See
Chapter 6, Section 2.) His recent record indicates
a minimum of alterations in symmetrical shape-flow,
with lengthening most prominent and occasional
hollowing. In asymmetrical shape-flow, widening is

rare, but the tendency to bulge and shorten remains. Widening may be replaced by rhythms of alternating "sideways" and "across-the-body" directions and by a similar, but less pronounced, tendency to spread and to enclose. An absorption of shape-flow attributes into the ego-controlled patterns of shaping makes Charlie less dependent on mood changes and more capable of developing deep relationships. Charlie's ability to be attentive and to explore, long impaired by his neurotic development, is beginning to show signs of recovery. In precursors of effort and directions, all patterns, needed for learning in a focused way, are now available to him. In the related patterns of effort and shaping in space, he still suffers from a constriction of functioning due to the severity of his superego (see postural patterns in directness and spreading p. 173 and Ch. 6, section IV.)

Both maturation and improvement of family conditions played a role in the easing of Nancy's relative retardation in development. Nevertheless, her tendency to use oral-sadistic rhythms in excess persists. Her late maturation expresses itself in her exaggerated use of differentiated rhythms, with mixed rhythms constituting a bit less than one-third of her rhythm-repertoire. The persistence of pathology can also be seen in the fact that even in her scanty mixed rhythms, "sadistic" components are more frequent than "libidinal" (p.131). Symmetrical shape-flow is considerably reduced in frequency-- the result of excessive stabilization. Nancy's body-attitude is dictated by her imitation of her father's neck position and by an eneven growth of limbs. Like a youngster in prepuberty (Kestenberg & Robbins, 1975), she extends her limbs by symmetrical and asymmetrical lengthening. Her inability to pay attention and her fiddling are still counteracted by a stabilization in bound flow, which has become quite noticeable in her thighs and calves. When she fiddles Nancy's staccato movements are still in evidence, but a great deal of her old abruptness has been subdued and converted into a tendency to accelerate. Although there are only a few postural patterns in her effort-repertoire, those that occur are loaded to a very high degree (59% load factor). When highly motivated, Nancy excels in tasks requiring indirectness, strength and acceleration. In this choice, she appears to be influenced by her father's effort-proclivities. Perhaps, the overstabilization of her shape-flow has retarded the development of shaping in planes in postural patterns. In clinical terms, we would say that Nancy has remained in a shell of aloneness and has not developed constant relationships, which would be governed by her ego-ideal.

I have selected several features of the newest profiles of Glenda, Charlie and Nancy to highlight some of the insight that can be gained about the influence of maturation and environmental influences on inborn and early rhythmic patterns. Perhaps, the questions that emerge can summarize best the gist of my findings:

Is maturation used to the best advantage of the child when the environment supports the maturational trend? If maturation and parents or educators, or both, reinforce patterns incompatible with original, innate preferences, are we to expect a neurotic development?

Are shape-flow and shaping more subject to external influences than tension-flow and efforts? We believe this to be so, but have to study it further. Do growth patterns influence shape-flow tendencies, so that lengthening is favored in growth periods and widening is favored in "feminine" phases. Does the stabilization of body-shape not only decrease symmetrical shape-changes, but also the selection of dimensional attributes?

CHAPTER 3

EARLY MANIFESTATIONS OF DISTURBED DEVELOPMENT
DUE TO CLASHES BETWEEN THE RHYTHMS OF INFANT AND MOTHER

A "good enough mother" (Winnicott, 1957) helps
create the baby's "average expectable environment"
(Hartmann, 1939) by empathizing with the child's needs
and creating in him a feeling of trust. Beginning with
this longitudinal study, and in the course of comparing
movement profiles of other mothers and their babies, we
have found that attunement in tension-flow is a good
measure of empathy, and that adjustment in shape-flow
is a good measure of mutual trust (Kestenberg & Buelte,
1977 a, b).

When the attunement is so complete that maternal
rhythms become indistinguishable from those of the
child, the fusion between them fosters a blissful state
of narcissism which becomes the basis for omnipotence
and aggrandizement rather than empathy (Kohut, 1971). In
average development, the attunement of maternal and infantile tension-flow rhythms comes to a peak in the early
oral phase and begins to decline with the onset of sepa-
ration-individuation (Mahler, 1968). When mother and
child each have a good correspondence (affinity) between
their own tension- and shape-flow rhythms, an attunement
in tension-flow between them automatically produces a
mutual adjustment in shape-flow.

Early attunement depends not only on maternal synchronization and equalization of tension-flow rhythms,
but also on the infant's capacity to modify his rhythms
in the service of a function. A mutually acceptable,
but inappropriate, use of rhythms leads to functional
disturbances. For instance, if mother and child both
prefer "phallic" to "oral" rhythms and use them during
nursing, they reinforce the mother's jumpiness and the
child's tendency to take big gulps, which brings on
choking or regurgitation. The attunement between mother
and baby must be function-oriented to be adaptive.

Adjustment in shape-flow does not mean that maternal
and infantile breathing must be synchronized, except when
it serves a circumscribed, shared activity. Through her
breathing, the caretaker helps the newborn to regularize
his own breathing, especially during nursing. Most important in this respect is the dimensional adjustment.
When breathing is synchronized and equalized, but proceed
in divergent planes, function may be considerably disturbed. During suckling, the baby's chest and arms widen

20

and there is some bulging, followed by narrowing with a bit of hollowing. His mother will harmonize with this rhythm of shape-flow by adjusting her chest and holding her arm in the horizontal plane, in which the baby alternately gains more room exhaling and comes closer to the nipple inhaling. If the mother would lengthen instead of widen at the same time as the baby inhales and widens, her nipple would pull away from him just at the time when he is ready to pump it for another swallow of milk. Giving the baby room for growing and shrinking is not only a matter of timing, but also the result of kinesthetic identification with the baby's dimensional shape-changes. By sharing the plane of shape-changes, mother and child develop a trust, based on a mutuality of fitting together.

When a mother attunes to the baby's tension-flow and adjusts to his shape-flow without consideration of optimal functioning, the immature or vulnerable baby does not have a chance to improve his survival skills. It is the task of the caretaker to teach the infant to choose appropriate rhythms; she not only must attune to him, but she must also teach him to attune to her. There are various degrees and modes of attunement and adjustment, but they are all based on the principle of affinity between related patterns (see chapter 6, section III). Not all attunement and adjustment is beneficial to development and not all clashes are detrimental (Kestenberg, 1975). Complete attunement, based on a synchronization of identical attributes and rhythms promotes sameness and a symbiotic attachment which exceeds the dual unity (described by Mahler, 1968) for the young nursling and his mother. When such an attunement is extreme and persists, it delays differentiation.

Partial clashing between rhythms may be a necessary preamble to retraining the child in the service of a function. For instance, a mother of a gulping nursling who uses "oro-phallic" rather than "oral" rhythms may--with success--rock him in an "oral" rhythm to induce his attunement to her and improve his suckling. Some forms of clashing are not based on an incompatibility of patterns, but rather on a failure to achieve sameness. For instance, a baby may use a "phallic" rhythm while kicking his legs. Playing with him, his mother may use a similar intensity, developed abruptly, but may also introduce a short period of even flow at the height of the tension. The rhythm will be changed, but the new attribute will not clash with the others, especially when the baby is receptive to moving with "oral-sadistic" biting rhythms, mixed with "phallic" rhythms. The mother will be adding novelty and will be enhancing the child's excitement rather than disturbing him. Quite different would be the situation

Early Manifestation

if even flow of long duration (a feature of the "anal-
sadistic" rhythm) was used by the mother of a wiggling,
twisting baby. Unless a compromise was formed immediately, the ensuing clash would quickly become a conflict
between mother and child.

Clashing intensely, without or with little attunement through the modification of opposing rhythms, or
clashing in more than one pattern, strains the child's
capacity to accommodate and may lead to an inhibition
and restriction of function.

Some children attune and adjust better to their
fathers or grandmothers than to their mothers. When, in
such cases, mother goes to work, the child may begin to
flourish with a more compatible caretaker. We assume
that early clashes lead to conflicts, but cannot agree
that the temporary removal of the incompatible mother
will do more than ameliorate the problem. It is our
experience that a child who clashes with his mother is
more clingy than one who lives in harmony with her, and
more afraid to lose her than one who feels her empathy
and can trust her. For some years now, we are developing methods of retraining mothers and babies to help them
develop the best possible attunement and adjustment. A
child may be greatly disturbed by the preponderant rhythm
of a sibling who has a different temperament or is en-
trenched in an "opposite" developmental phase. A house-
keeper or day-worker who clashes with the baby can be
replaced by a more compatible person, but parents and
siblings need to learn to get along by attuning, which
leads to better understanding, and by adjusting, to make
the family a reliable respondent to the child's styles of
relating. Mothers learn to help children of different
ages to attune and adjust to others. This usually takes
some time before it can be accomplished. Some children
who clash with their mothers or siblings early, eventuall
learn to accept the foreign rhythmicity; others accept it
at times, partially or under protest. Consequently, one
sometimes sees, juxtaposed, conflicts with the mother and
identification with her, a constellation which leads to
early internalization of conflict.

The differences in the result of early clashes are
not only dependent on their nature, their source, their
sporadic or all-pervasive occurrence, but also on the
differences in patterns of organization.

Because of the biphasic organization which
characterized Glenda's temperament, she was able to
attune to her mother in one phase and continue with
her preferred rhythm in the second phase of an
activity. Because her mother primed her early to
enjoy anal rhythms, Glenda became more accommodating

and achieved enough stability to enhance her autonomy in the second year of life. A similar stabilization, based on the confluence between attunement
to the mother and maturation, could be observed in
the middle phase of Glenda's pregnancy--a time when
anal rhythms usually increase (Kestenberg, 1976).
Whenever maturation had the effect of making her
tension-flow rise more gradually than before,
Glenda went through periods of better attunement
with her mother. However, not until the middle
phase of her pregnancy did she develop enough
shortening (sinking in the middle) to allow for a
good mirroring of her mother's body attitude. Adjusting to her in shape-flow, she began to widen as
well, but could do this only in the periphery of her
body. Depressed and feeling small, as compared with
her mother, Glenda began to shorten, not only by
sinking, but also by hunching her shoulders up, by
putting her hand to her face and by dropping her
head. She could still pull herself out of the dol-
drums by lengthening, both symmetrically and asymmetrically, an attitude which expressed the renewal
of her optimism.

Retrospectively, we can see that there must have
been considerable clashing in shape-flow rhythms
between mother and baby Glenda. From the start,
mother would fluctuate, praising the child when she
fulfilled her own thwarted aspirations, but begrudg-
ing her the ability to comfort herself and forget
her troubles. When Glenda needed comforting, mother
would apply her own method of doing it by widening
and thus expressing her generosity. Glenda did not
seem to be able to adjust to this method too well.
She tended to feel constricted and used to combat
the constriction by literally lifting herself up.
Perhaps an important source of satisfaction to
Glenda's mother was the child's long and narrow
frame - a shape more in keeping with the image of
a phallus than her own. However, she felt deprived
because of Glenda's inability to steadily give of
herself and become voluble by widening like her
mother. Glenda could widen peripherally, but even
that was shortlived and was quickly replaced by
lengthening. Glenda's periodic attunement and her
periodic attempts to adjust to her mother made it
possible for her to function by dividing her conflicts in a shorter or longer temporal sequence.
The biphasic solution--akin to doing and undoing--
made her more dependent on external circumstances
and passing states, and diminished her capacity to
internalize punitive codes.

Early Manifestation

   Clashes between maternal and infantile rhythms may not be as evident in bottle-fed as they are in breast-fed babies. Some babies hold their bottle very early and need hardly any cuddling during nutritive sucking. As long as they are held securely with the bottle held for them properly, most babies need not depend on their mothers' fine attunement in tension-flow and adjustment in shape-flow. During breast feeding, clashing in rhythms disturbs function and the experience is not satisfactory for either mother or child. Many mothers do not know why they prefer bottle feeding to nursing; they simply experience a reluctance, which, on closer scrutiny, proves to be a lack of confidence in their own ability to empathize and to feel trust. When clashing is very tedious, mothers will resort to prop-feeding. Problems are avoided in this manner, but they become manifest during the feeding of solids. The mistiming and misshaping of spoonfuls, given to the baby, reflects permanent or temporary clashes between mother and child. Self-feeding, which arises from the mirroring of maternal movements, may be delayed. Some passive infants learn to sit through feedings in almost total immobility, holding their hands up and sideways, in order not to interfere with maternal actions. Inhibitions and restriction of movement is the price paid for acceding instead of clashing. Those who refuse solids and want to be left alone with their bottle learn to avoid clashes by withdrawal.

   Charlie's early ability to modify qualities of tension, in response to the excitement generated by his mother, revealed itself in his early dialogue with her (vol 1., p. 15 of first paper of this series; 1965). In attunement with his mother's preferred phallic rhythms, he would become less gradual and would incorporate abrupt and frequent flow fluctuations into his basic pattern of excitation. There was a correspondence in shape-flow as well, as each of them was bulging towards the other as if they could bridge the distance between them by a change of shape. These periods of excitement were relatively infrequent. Soon, his mother ceased to hold him for bottle-feeding and he began to hold his own bottle early. His capacity to modify his preferential rhythms came to an end when, at the age of seven months, he had to sit in the kitchen where he was confronted by too many divergent stimuli. He was not only bombarded by his mother's but also by his siblings' phallic rhythms, and these were not always synchronized. A clash in shape-flow and directions aggravated the situation. Charlie shortened by sliding downward, widened and turned sideways while his mother lengthened and towered over him, standing in a narrow stance, some

distance from him, and bringing the spoon forward
and down to his mouth. Charlie did not look up,
but stared ahead, sometimes turning his gaze to
the two toddlers who crowded around him and seemed
to bulge towards him. The spoon came to Charlie
as a surprise; he turned away from it sideways and
even backward, in his gradual mode of tension-flow.
The spoon followed him abruptly and Charlie responded by becoming more and more intense. Eventually, he would cry and would work himself up to a
very high degree of excitation. Returned to his
crib he was content; he turned to his bottle and
drank from it in his own gradual, deliberate manner. He played with his toes and reached for objects when they were held in front of him for a
long enough time. Charlie could modify his rhythms,
up to a certain point, beyond which he asserted himself and withdrew. When he was a toddler, he insisted that his mother adjust to him by sitting down
to hold him. In latency, his insistence on retaining his own mode of functioning led to clashes with
his mother and his teachers. In adolescence, he
began to tower over her and look down on her. He
began to make sarcastic remarks about his teachers.
The influx of oral-sadistic rhythms has persisted,
but in keeping with his original preferences, inner-
genital rhythms exceed the phallic, especially in
mixed rhythms. However, his original tendency to
widen has been replaced by frequent lengthening.
He has taken on some of his mother's qualities, such
as abruptness and acceleration.

The early clashes left an indelible imprint on
Charlie's learning habits, defenses and coping patterns. Conflicts developed early and their internalization resulted in a restriction of his explor-
atory curiosity and a reduction of his attention
span. We wonder how much of Charlie's integrative
capacity has been spent on maintaining a neurotic
organization. We are reminded of his early capacity
to absorb his mother's preferred rhythms (probably
"phallic" and "oral-sadistic") and his subsequent
need to withdraw rather than compromise - at a time
when his teething became acute. We witnessed then
the results of clashing and interference with functioning, which derailed Charlie's integrative capacity into the service of inhibition, a very early
precursor of the superego.

Charlie's early clashes predictably led to conflicts,
at first external and soon internalized. Since I have
studied his development I have come across similar cases
of early infantile clashing which led to early pathology
and to a severity of the superego.

Early Manifestation

A delay in structure formation can be expected where too many flow fluctuations and an innate predisposition to disorganization is met by measures promoting rigidity and limpness. Rigidity enhances a stable body-shape early, precluding adjustment to other people's shapes and the developmental progression of dimensional factors of shape-flow. Limpness is associated with an abnormal state of consciousness, expressed in movement through neutral flow in tension and shape. The inert, limp, shapeless body can neither attune nor adjust. In states of abnormally prolonged or all too frequent neutral flow (see p. 61), the organism loses its elasticity and plasticity. The caretaking mother needs to revitalize the baby by touching, massaging and stimulating him. If he alternates between these abnormal states and equally abnormal states of disorganized excitement, she too may alternate between overstimulating him and leaving him alone.

Nancy, in her infancy, alternated between undue excitement, rigidity and limpness. In her home life she was alternately overstimulated and isolated with a propped bottle. Unlike Charlie, she would become rigid in her body and exaggerate her partial stabilization until she became immobile. When prevented from self-feeding, she clutched spoons to stabilize herself. Before she could stand, mother enticed her to "dance" to what seemed to be a violent kind of rhythm. It is difficult to speak of attunement or adjustment in Nancy's case. One can recognize a tendency to sameness and to mirroring of the mother which persists today. Her development is not yet completed. Her ego and superego functions developed late and the latter is based only on the internalization of punitive tendencies. Internalization of ego ideals lags behind (see Nancy's lack of postural shaping in her profile).

In appraising the effect of early clashes between mother and child, we have to distinguish between disturbances of isolated functions, due to clashes, and disturbances of general characteristics, caused by an incompatibility of temperaments. Charlie's refusals to eat or reach are examples of isolated inhibitions, comparable to the "symptoms" of an older child. The withdrawal to the "hinterland", where there is peace, is a generalized attitude, designed to safeguard Charlie's temperament. Preferences for certain rhythms, seen in short periods of observation, are also in evidence over longer spans of time, in diurnal "excitation-gratification-relaxation-rest cycles". One can see a parallel between rhythms occuring during activities giving functional pleasure, and the periodicity of repeated "need-discharge-rest cycles". Thus, Glenda not only used abruptly rising and falling rhythms of tension-flow, which were followed by short rests, but she also engaged in short period of nutritive sucking, which were followed by relatively short rests. Charlie not only preferred gradually rising, intense and very gradually subsiding tension changes in his play actions and during feeding, but his whole behavior-day was characterized by sequences of very gradual arousals, long periods of intense enjoyment or intense frustration (subsiding very gradually), and periods of rest--most probably in neutral flow. Nancy's behavior-day was as irregular as her short, erratic rhythms of tension-flow. She sucked voraciously, became frustrated very quickly and resumed her excitement quickly, becoming rigid in the process. What at first was described as a complete relaxation, seems, retrospectively, more like limpness.

Surveying these children's development, and comparing their total behavior today with that of their early infancy, we detect that regardless of the changes in the ratio of their tension-flow and shape-flow rhythms, and regardless of the contributions of more advanced movement patterns, their basic temperament has remained the same. It is difficult to appraise the cycles of their behavior-days, but one can be guided by the changes that occur during much longer periods of time. Glenda is still given to periodic, impulsive decisions, and does not take sufficient time to weigh the consequences of the changes she institutes in her life. Her mother still complains that Glenda starts many things which she does not finish, as she used to do as an infant. Charlie still takes a very long time before he changes his mind, and he still withdraws when he reaches the limit of his endurance. His mother's main complaint is that he is not getting around to making up the one test which would complete his high school requirements. For some time now, Charlie has contemplated passing the omitted test so that he can enroll in college. In the meantime, he has devoted himself to finding and furnishing his own place to live. He gets along well with his mother, but he visits her only when he is good and ready; and she is learning, at last, to accept his way of doing things. The greatest change has·occurred in Nancy, who is progressing in her drive, ego and superego development. She is less limp now and much more lively. However, despite her progress, she has remained erratic. She interrupts one idea by another, working and enrolling in college, going out with a boyfriend (who is "not a boyfriend") and disorganizing all her endeavors by adopting her sister's interest in witches and after-life.

Early Manifestation

We have seen the influence of clashes between maternal and infantile rhythms of tension-flow and shape-flow on early development. Even more conspicuous is the long-term clashing in temperaments which could be seen in the cases of Glenda and Charlie. The attempt to change Nancy by isolating her from the rest of her family in the beginning of her first year did not alter her temperament, as it is still evident today. Rather, it merely retarded her development. However, in Nancy's case, there is an essential similarity between her, her mother and especially her grandmother. In Glenda's case, there was a resemblance between her temperament and that of her grandmother, and Charlie's temperament did not seem to differ from that of his father. These are the familial roots of temperament.

Little is known about the somatic (perhaps neuro-hormonal) processes underlying temperamental differences. Whatever they are, they seem to be superordinated over the distribution of rhythms on which drive discharge is based. There seems to be a relationship between tempera-ment and preferred discharge forms, but the nature of this relationship is still to be explored. We can say that an early clash of temperaments between mother and child complicates the development of relationships. Sameness in temperament enhances the qualities that go into "getting along". Diversity may lead to escape or withdrawal, without necessarily diminishing the depth of feelings between love objects.

Clashing between maternal and infantile tension-flow and shape-flow rhythms are not uncommon in early infancy, but clashing of temperaments is rarely as pronounced as was seen in the cases of Glenda and especially Charlie. To delineate an infant's temperament we shall have to study not only the observable movement patterns and their distribution in hourly periods, but we will need to ex-tend observations to twenty-four-hour periods and longer. In addition, we will have to pay attention to the pos-sibility that there are preferences for certain states of arousal, which can be seen in infancy and may be re-tained in adulthood. The connection between states of arousal and tension changes--both mediated by the reticular zone--need to be explored, and a method of comparing infantile and adult states has to be devised before clashes between temperaments of infant and care-taker can be meaningfully appraised.

In summary, I can confirm that early clashes between mother and child are most frequently based on a lack of attunement in tension-flow and/or adjustment in shape-flow. Too close an attunement may forebode too close an attachment, which may interfere with differentiation. In normal development, it is the task of the mother to help the child learn the matching of appropriate rhythms to specific discharge modes and areas of functioning. Partial clashing between mother and child can create a basis for compromise and for the acceptance of patterns which the mother chooses as best suited for differentiated activities. Clashes between temperaments must be studied by observations of behavior-days and even longer periods of time.

CHAPTER 4

LATER BEHAVIOR WHICH CAN BE DERIVED FROM
MOTOR RHYTHMS

In the beginning of this study, all references to
rhythms pertained to "tension-flow-rhythms" which were
classified and named later. We know now that all motion
factors can be organized in rhythms, and intrinsic to
each rhythm are the attributes and elements of the
motion factors involved. Movement is composed of many
interlapping and coordinated rhythms. In tension-flow
rhythms the attributes of tension-flow are subsumed under the heading of "intensity factors"; shape-flow
rhythms repeat and alternate attributes of motion which
are referred to as "dimensional factors". Rhythms of
precursors of effort and effort consist of repetitions of
their respective elements (Laban, 1960). A simple effort
rhythm can be seen in hammering in which lightness and
strength alternate. Other advanced, ego-controlled
motion factors, such as shaping our space in directions
and planes, are also subject to their own rhythmicity
which varies from individual to individual and from one
functional activity to another. The interplay of rhythms
of all these movement qualities cannot be given full
justice until we can devise means of simultaneous consecutive notations of all action patterns in a given
phrase. At this time we are capable only of notating
consecutive changes and repetitions in tension-flow and
in shape-flow design. The classification and interpretation of tension-flow rhythms has developed further through
the years and we have begun to correlate these rhythms
with behavior. (See Section I of this chapter.) A classification of rhythms of shape-flow-design has not yet
progressed beyond its early stages. Preliminary data of
their correlation with behavior will be discussed in
Section II of this chapter.

Section I

Tension-Flow Rhythms and Behavior
———————————————————————————————

Rhythms of tension-flow consist of regular or
irregular repetitions of certain units which are characterized by specific sequences of qualities of tension.
Notations of tension-flow-changes reveal specific rhythmic units which can be recognized by their design on
paper. Werner (1948, p. 70) explained the recognition
of these units by our capacity for physiognomic perception. He reproduced three linear drawings which, in an
investigation by Krauss, were correlated with the emotional content of given words. It is interesting to
note that two of the designs are identical with our
notation of "oral-sadistic" and "phallic-sadistic"
rhythms respectively, and the third looks like a mixed
"phallic-oral" rhythm. In appraising these similarities
we must remember that our notations are representations
of changes of tension and cannot be translated into
specific emotions. However, there is a correlation
between specific rhythms and the drive discharge modes
for which they are suited, and there is a correlation
between temperament, affect and tension-flow attributes.

Perhaps a scrutiny of the relation between rhythms
and their intrinsic tension-flow attributes will shed
some light on the complexity of the correlations we
postulate.

"Oral" rhythmic units (⌒ or ⌣) are represented
in half-circles. They are drawn above the neutral line
when their flow is free and below when it is bound.
Sucking consists of repetitions of soft (arched) alternations between free and bound flow. When sucking in-
tensifies to smacking or gulping, a quality of intensity
of tension is added, but the sinus curve continues:

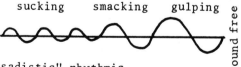

sucking   smacking   gulping

"Oral-sadistic" rhythmic
snapping units are represented in half-squares (⋀ or ⋁).
They too, alternate from free to bound flow, but the
transition between free and bound is sharp. Bound flow
is experienced as inhibition (tightness) and free flow
as release. The pleasure in sucking is derived from the
release in free flow and the smoothness of reversals from
free to bound flow and vice versa. The snapping, biting
rhythm is frequently used by the infant to alleviate teeth-

ing pain. Its free flow provides for the relief-pleasure, associated with biting and the sharpness of reversals, added to the constraint in bound flow, accentuates the unplea ure also associated with biting. The "oral" rhythm with i smooth renewal of free flow becomes a model for continuity and sameness. The "oral-sadistic" rhythm with its emphasi on sharp reversals and bound flow reduces the smoothness o continuity and introduces a foreboding of discontinuity.

The release of tension in free flow facilitates the transmission of impulses and, thus, serves the aim of the erotic drive (Freud, 1920). Bound flow, which in- hibits impulses, is likely to serve the aim of the aggressive drive. We hypothesize that "libidinal" rhythms, such as sucking, must have at least one aggres- sive component to produce a contrast between binding and release that is the essence of pleasure (Freud, 1917, p. 160). The binding of flow itself is usually the only non-libidinal factor in sucking. It is coun- teracted by the smooth transformation of bound into free flow and vice versa. We hypothesize that "sadistic" rhythms contribute many more aggressive components than do "libidinal", pleasurable and pain-free rhythms. The pleasure-pain of snapping, via a sharp transformation of free into bound flow and vice versa, appears to be the prototype of affects released through sadistic discharge forms.

We can now begin to distinguish between the pleasant feeling in the release of free flow or the constrained feeling in the binding of flow and the pleasure aspects of the rhythmic alternations of these qualities. A feel- ing of ease and its polarity, a feeling of unease, are the simplest affective patterns representing the basic dichotomy between life-giving and aggressive drives. Smoothness and sharpness of reversals are further refine- ments which trigger off the basic qualities of predominant pleasure and pleasure-pain experiences, respectively.

More advanced "oral-sadistic" biting units (⎽⏌⎼
or ⎽⏌⎽) are characterized by an attribute of tension- flow which adds another dimension to expressions of ag- gression: a quality of holding the intensity of binding or releasing on an even level. The short duration of this attribute of tension-flow gives the biter a "fore- taste" of endurance and maintenance of sameness which become pronounced in "anal-sadistic" straining rhythms. Biting appears to be a small scale model for the pleasure- unpleasure quality of holding. The principal character- istic of biting is evenness of tension of short duration. Adjustment of tension levels is the principal character-

istic of twisting "anal" rhythms which can be best seen
in the contractions of the anal sphincter. While holding permits a longer contact with an object or an organ, twisting (~~~~~~~~~~) is an initiator
of play, whose prototype is the response of the sphincter
to external stimuli such as wiping. Its closing and
opening style is coordinated with small changes in the
intensity of tension. The "anal" rhythm is pleasurable
by virtue of its smooth variations of low, but uneven intensities of tension and release. The attributes of tension-flow adjustment and low intensity, intrinsic to the
"anal" rhythm, can be correlated with such affective qualities as the seeking of change (a motor response to uniform
stimuli) and the delicate refinement of small nuances of
feeling tones. Their combination in "anal" rhythms underlies the joy of rhythmic playfulness. We note that
the two principal attributes of this system (adjustment
of level and low intensity) serve the aims of erotic
drives. Sameness-promoting even flow is more likely to
be subservient to aggression. The most common form of a
straining "anal-sadistic" rhythm ⌣‾‾‾‾⌣ displays

the attributes of high intensity of tension, with a prolonged holding of an even level of intensity in bound
flow. These qualities are correlated with intense feelings, with endurance or persistence, and with caution,
respectively. They are all used in the service of aggressive aims. Combined, they account for the quality of
holding back. However, free flow may initiate or terminate the "anal-sadistic" rhythmic unit, and there is enough
variability in flow, in the rate of change, in duration,
and in intensity to account for an admixture of "libidinal"
attributes to its predominantly aggressive components.

    "Urethral" rhythmic units are characterized by a
gradual ascent or descent of tension in linear or
vibrating succession of tension changes. The predominant attribute of this rhythm regardless of its variations ‾‾‾‾‾‾\/‾‾‾ is a gradual

rise or fall of tension and release. Graduality introduces a quality of pleasant leisure. In combination with
free and decreasing bound flow it is experienced as pleasure in mobility with the overtone of "letting go" or
"running out". Variations of the "urethral-sadistic"
"run-stop-go" rhythmic units encompass graduality

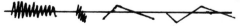

or abruptness, but their common feature is a sharp reversal
of free into bound flow. The attribute of abruptness underlies such basic reactions as impulsivity or quickness
of responses. Combined with sharp reversals it accentuate
the aggressive aims of such impulses as "shooting out".
Free flow becomes the source of pleasure in the initiation
of "going". In a variant form of the "urethral-sadistic"
rhythm, graduality combines with sharpness of tension-flow
reversals to produce a sequence of pleasure-unpleasure in
the experience of "run-stop-go".

Undulant "inner-genital" rhythms consist of very
gradually rising and falling tension and release, with
smooth, sometimes almost imperceptible transitions from

free to bound flow ⁓⁓⁓⁓⁓⁓⁓⁓⁓⁓⁓⁓⁓ . In con-

trast to the "anal-sadistic" and "urethral" rhythms they
vary little and always preserve the appearance of extremely elongated "oral" rhythmic units. Their low intensity
and graduality reflects subtleness of feelings and leisure
liness, respectively. Combined with one another and with
free or bound flow, as well as with smoothness of tension-
flow reversals, they provide the motor substrate of
pleasure derived from waves of excitation traveling
through the body. The high intensity of tension achieved
very gradually in "swaying inner-genital-sadistic" types

rhythm introduces ⟋‾‾‾‾‾‾‾‾

an attribute, serving aggressive aims and perceived as
intenseness. The sequence of gradually evolving high
intensity in bound and free flow is experienced in the
unpleasure-pleasure range of prolonged expulsive contractions and relaxations.

The "jumping phallic" rhythm is primarily characterized by an abrupt rise and fall of tension and release, with a smooth transition between them. The additional attribute of high intensity is not obligatory, but
phallic spurts in low intensity (⌐∿⌐) are seen infre-

quently. The combination of abruptness with smooth reversals accounts for the predominantly pleasurable experience for which the metaphors of "flying" or "para-
chuting" are most appropriate.

The "leaping phallic-sadistic" rhythm ⋀⋀⋀⋀⋀⋀⋀⋀

combines abruptness with sharp reversals from free to bound flow and vice versa. The predominance of qualities used in aggressive discharge forms is counteracted only by the pleasurable release into free flow. This combination accounts for the explosive nature of phallic-sadistic gratification.

The detailed account of qualities of rhythms helped us to discover that attributes of tension-flow are not the sole determinants of differences between rhythmic units. A sharp or smooth reversal from free into bound flow and vice versa should not be confused with an abrupt or gradual rise and fall of tension.[4]) All "libidinal" type rhythms share the quality of smooth reversal of flow. Sharp reversals characterize all "sadistic" type rhythms except the "anal-sadistic" and the "sadistic-inner-genital". These long-lasting rhythmic forms have a greater capacity to organize and subsume other rhythms into their course.

We can distinguish short and long rhythmic units. The short ones tend to repeat themselves more often than the long ones. Thus, oral and phallic discharge forms maintain continuity by oscillation. In a lesser measure, the same is true of anal and the vibratory urethral rhythms. A rise and fall of intensity may proceed with a minimum of flow changes or it can incorporate many small flow fluctuations into its course. The former account for steadiness of discharge, and the latter for playfulness, as observed in the use of anal rhythms, or restlessness, as noted in some activities performed with urethral rhythms.

We know of one more factor by which rhythms can be distinguished. Some pure rhythms are variable, as for instance, the "oral-sadistic"

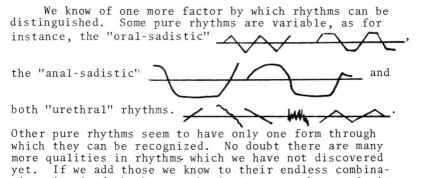

the "anal-sadistic" and both "urethral" rhythms.

Other pure rhythms seem to have only one form through which they can be recognized. No doubt there are many more qualities in rhythms which we have not discovered yet. If we add those we know to their endless combinations in mixed rhythms, we begin to grasp the complexity

---

[4]) Flow reversals must not be confused with reversals of direction in shape-flow-design, which can be sharp (angular) or smooth (rounded) (see section 2, p. 57).

of rhythmic discharge forms which - we believe - underlie the qualities of drives. Perhaps a survey of our three subjects' original and later preferences for certain tension-flow attributes and rhythms will illustrate the difficulties encountered in trying to correlate infants' rhythms with later behavior.

Glenda's original preference for "phallic" rhythms carried with it a predilection for abrupt changes of tension which often reached a high intensity of release in free flow. In the new-born nursery she stood out because of her ability to fling her legs up and initiate locomotion while supine. She would spend herself in such activities and would need a rest. Whether present from the beginning or added later, snapping "oral-sadistic" rhythms would frequently fill the inter-vals between flings. Biphasic functioning of this type permeated her behavior-day and could be noted during short periods of observation as well. She would become involved in an exciting activity in an abrupt fashion, and would pursue it briefly to give it up as abruptly as it started. After a short rest or a period of fiddling she would resume her carefree flings. At four, when her brother was born, she was flooded by "oral-sadistic" rhythms and "phallic" rhythms decreased. At the peak of the phallic phase "phallic-sadistic" rhythms became prominent while her biphasic functioning receded throughout the phallic phase. Instead, a quality of continuous excitement gave her behavior a frantic tinge.

During latency, she used "phallic" rhythms for play and fun and imbued her sedentary work, such as drawing, writing or cutting, with "snapping oral-sadistic" rhythms in which bound flow predominated. The sedentary work was encouraged by the mother, but Glenda appeared tortured while obeying her. It would have been more appropriate then to speak of "oral masochistic" patterning. At the end of her adoles-cence, Glenda still used a good many "phallic" rhy-thms which perpetuated her propensity for abrupt-ness. However, they were more noticeable in prepa-rations for and transitions to new phrases. High intensity was not favored, and "inner-genital" rhy-thms were almost as frequent as "phallic". During her pregnancy, "phallic" rhythms were outweighed by anal components in pure and by inner genital libid-inal in mixed rhythms. Throughout her development, Glenda responded to maturation and to her mother's influence by decreasing her abruptness in comparison with other attributes of her tension repertoire.

During latency, she became more patient and controlled, and used biphasic functioning to make a compromise between needs and external demands. Vivacious exclamations would be followed by lip-biting and fiddling--especially when her mother criticized her. We shall see in Chapter 6 how the preference for "phallic" rhythms influenced her choice of such ego-controlled defensive and coping mechanisms, as suddenness and acceleration, in making decisions.

It seems that Charlie's originally preferred rhythm could be classified as "inner-genital-sadistic". A placid baby, Charlie used so few flow fluctuations that he felt heavy in one's arms. Adjustment of tension levels was sometimes so minimal that it constituted an obstacle to attunement. His propensity for gradually evolving and gradually subsiding high tension and release was counteracted by the many abrupt flow-fluctuations imposed upon him by his siblings and his mother. When Charlie did absorb them into his prevailing organization, it made him look like a deliberate adult, temporarily engaged in play. In latency, his persistence in a gradual mode intensified his conflicts with his mother and teacher. Through a considerable reduction in intensity of tension, he now makes greater use of "libidinal inner-genital" rhythms. Due to a family crisis and illness, Charlie's vivacious mother has become more sedentary and subdued. Mother and son now share a preference for "libidinal inner-genital" rhythms. Charlie is still capable of integrating a variety of stimuli into a uniform experience. This helps him manage the many sarcastic, biting remarks which he utters, with great charm and within a generally good-natured attitude. However, his learning disturbance persists and his work suffers, not only because of his tendency to stare in neutral flow, but also because the early clashes between himself and his mother had been carried over into his work-patterns.

It is likely that Charlie's original strong predisposition for rhythms combining graduality with high intensity was the source of a persistent internal conflict (Freud, A., 1965). These two attributes have contradictory trends, the first towards passivity and the second towards activity (Kestenberg & Marcus, 1978). The resulting conflict diminished when a shift occurred from the "sadistic" to the "libidinal" "inner-genital" rhythm. By this time, his internalized conflicts were on the increase and he used his capacity to integrate and absorb to enforce his neurotic organization.

37

Later Behavior

Nancy, in her infancy, showed a prevalence of oral discharge forms which invaded and derailed others. Nancy's behavior was bizarre; she fell victim to an overwhelming amount of irregular flow fluctuations. A preponderance of sharp transitions from free to bound flow made her appear jerky. The early propping of the bottle became an aid in the achievement of partial stabilization through bound flow. Her harrassed mother, her deprived father and her siblings promoted a disorganization which matched or outdid Nancy's internal upheaval. Nancy responded to internal and external sources of over-stimulation by becoming rigid, unresponsive or limp. Her body attitude is still rigid and she still tends to become limp in her wrists, but inertia befalls her more often. "Oral-sadistic" rhythms are still excessive, but their influence is overshadowed by a combination of two "sadistic" rhythms (urethral-and phallic-sadistic). As a result, "sadistic" type rhythms exceed their "libidinal" counterparts both in pure and mixed rhythms. This is an ominous finding (see Nancy's profile, p. 131).

It is likely that Nancy's proclivity for disorganization was fostered by a preponderance of "sadistic" rhythms which, by virtue of their sharp reversals, tended to interrupt rather than amalgamate with others. Her early deprivation was caused by a combination of neglect and the insatiability of her needs. Because so many different rhythms interrupted one another it was extremely difficult to reconstruct her preferred rhythmic sequences and to interpret them. At twenty, Nancy has many "urethral-sadistic" rhythms which combine with "phallic-sadistic" rhythms. This may have been part of her original predilection. No doubt, family circumstances fostered it as well. Nancy's older brother was her competitor from the start. The only boy among girls, he succeeded in going to college while working. Just recently, Nancy confessed that she had wrecked her brother's bicycle and incurred his anger. Mindful that Nancy's development was delayed, and that she never reached a peak of the urethral and the phallic phases, we must consider that we are witnessing now not the results of a fixation or a regression, but a belated appearance of patterns which could not proceed at the appropriate maturational phases (Greenacre, 1954).

In summary, our study suggests that a variety of behaviors can be derived from early tension-flow rhythms. The originally preferred rhythms increase or decrease by attunement with the mother. An impulsive or lively baby

can calm down in a placid environment. The congenitally
preferred rhythms increase in the developmental phases in
which these patterns predominate. However, with increasing maturation, the role of rhythms in behavior changes.
For instance, Glenda's early use of "phallic" rhythms
underlaid her capacity to fling herself in early infancy;
in the phallic phase it enhanced her frequent jumping, and
in latency it contributed to the enjoyment of skilled gross
motor activities. In adolescence and early adulthood,
"phallic" rhythms made Glenda's transitions from one
action-phrase to the next particularly abrupt and impulsive.
She changed from one topic to another with the "Jack-in-
the-Box" quality of a phallic child. Once she has flung
herself into a new topic, she developed a theme, characterized by more gradual changes in tension-flow. During the
inner-genital orientation of her pregnancy (Kestenberg,
1976),"phallic" rhythms decreased. Such a relative reversal
occurs regularly in phases, in which rhythms, opposite to
those originally preferred, become abundant. However, the
original preference need not be eradicated.

More striking than the persistence of certain rhythms
in development is the persistence of their organization
into adulthood. Glenda's biphasic actions, Charlie's
capacity to integrate and Nancy's propensity for repetition and immobilization exemplify the carry over of predominant modes of organization from infancy into adulthood. The respective organizations reveal themselves in
current behavior in such a way that Glenda makes rash
decisions which she only partially carries out; Charlie
absorbs things slowly, but succeeds in putting them together into such ideas as creating his own business, and;
Nancy repeats her ideas without self-criticism and can
function only in simple, repetitive jobs which require
sedentary activity.

Section II

Rhythms of Shape-Flow Design and Behavior

Each motor pattern is repeated in shorter or longer
intervals. In this sense, all movement is rhythmic. If
we were to write changes in each pattern in the same
manner as we notate tension changes, we might be able
to see the formal representations of rhythms in all
patterns. However, as of today, we can only notate ten-

sion-flow rhythms and rhythms of shape-flow-design.[5]

The most basic apparatus for interaction is the rhythmic alternation and repetition of centrifugal and centripetal movements, with pathways leading away from the body and back towards it. The former can move from "near-space" (near the body) through "intermediate space" and into "reach space", beyond which is the general space. The latter move towards the body and into the body from the "reach space" through the "intermediate space" and into the "near space". Pathways of centrifugal and centripetal movements form designs which are repeated in regular and irregular intervals. These design-units (see Illustration 1) vary from activity to activity, and from person to person.

Illustration 1

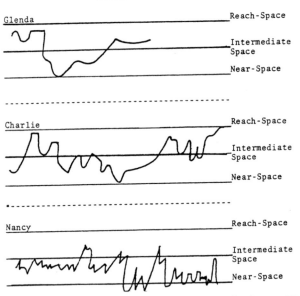

Illustration 1. Representative samples of shape-flow-design rhythms from the latest profiles of Glenda, Charlie and Nancy.

---

[5] The notation of shape-flow-design rhythms was developed by the author and Forrestine Paulay, who, at the time, was collaborating with Lomax and Bartenieff (1967) in their choreometric study of ethnic groups.

They are also dependent on maturation. For instance, small arcs or triangles in near space are characteristic of young infants. Children in latency are most comfortable in the intermediate space and mid-adolescents like to move in reach-space. Cultural influences affect shape-flow design rhythms more than any other single pattern. However, congenital preferences for certain design-rhythms can be noticed at birth.

We have not been able to classify shape-flow-design rhythms in a manner similar to tension-flow rhythms. We score attributes of design rhythms as:

Loops or lines

Low or high amplitudes

Smooth or sharp reversals of direction [6]
and refer to them as "design factors".

A retrospective appraisal of design factors can be attempted for all three subjects of the study, but only in Glenda's case was I able to reconstruct a typical design rhythm characteristic of her neonatal flinging stunts (see Illustration 2).

Illustration 2

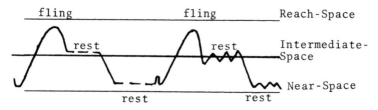

Illustration 2. Reconstruction of Glenda's shape-flow-design as a neonate, flinging her legs upward and sideways. Whether the rest periods were characterized by immobility (broken lines) or by small, jerky movements cannot be established from the description in the record.

---

[6] A belated insight prompts me to revise the terms applied to attributes of shape-flow-design. Rather than "smooth" and "sharp", the terms "angular" and "rounded" are more appropriate.

Later Behavior

As shown in Illustration 2, Glenda tended to alternate between small and high amplitudes, the latter extending her movement into reach space. She used rounded reversals for flinging motions, but the jerkiness of her
small motions was produced by angular reversals. In this
example, she preferred linear movement to loops or undu-
lations.

It is difficult at first to distinguish between tension-flow and shape-flow-design rhythms. By superimposing
the schematic representations of both rhythms, one can
recognize the differences between them which may be
otherwise overlooked (see Illustration 3).

Illustration 3

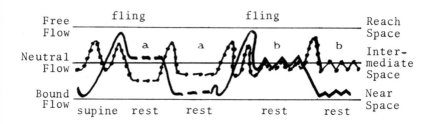

Illustration 3. Glenda's neonatal flinging, schematically
represented in shape-flow-design- (___) and tension-flow
(••••)-notations.

In Illustration 3 the smoothness and sharpness of
reversals from free to bound flow and vice versa correspond to the manner in which directions are reversed in
shape-flow-design. However, reversals in flow need not
be accompanied by reversals in direction. We note that as
Glenda's flinging proceeds, free flow decreases, bound flow
ensues and free flow is revived once more before the fling
is completed. Free flow and centrifugal motions, and bound
flow and centripetal motions frequently go together, but
their correspondence is not obligatory. Three phallic
units occur during one fling into reach space and another
before the rest period in the supine position. Bound flow
remains on an even keel during the immobility of the rest

periods (a). Jerky motions of small amplitude (b) have an identical form to "oral-sadistic" type rhythms. A similar correspondence between tension- and design-rhythms can be seen elsewhere during sucking motions. There is a certain correspondence between attributes of the two rhythms, and sometimes--as in "oral" rhythms--their notations can be identical. Yet, there is a basic difference between them. One notates tension changes and the other notates the changes in the nature of pathways of movement.

While tension-changes reflect the alterations in needs and in feelings of danger and safety, the changes in pathways express shades of feelings of relatedness, in the area of clinging and seeking (Hermann, 1963; Balint, 1959). Rhythms of tension-flow, as representatives of needs and drives, serve basic satisfactions which cannot be accomplished without the mediation of satisfying objects. Shape-flow-design is the apparatus via which the space between oneself and others can be traversed. We postulate that there are typical rhythms of relatedness which correspond to, but need not be identical with, rhythms of need-satisfaction. In the absence of models for rhythms of relatedness, we have not been able to classify shape-flow-design rhythms as we classified tension-flow rhythms. We can correlate behavior with design attributes, but are not at all certain that the original predilections for such attributes remain. A few examples will serve to illustrate the complexity of shape-flow-design interpretations.

Glenda, in her infancy and childhood, had a predilection for rounded reversals. She was abrupt but not jerky. Her movements became still rounder in inner-genital phases, and this corresponded to a more refined approach to people (see Illustration 1a). As an infant, Charlie changed directions rarely and when he did, the reversals were rounded. He preferred to move in small amplitudes. When stimulated by his mother, he strained forward, oscillating rapidly, and his reversals became not only more frequent but also more angular. During adolescence, Charlie's amplitudes increased considerably. He lost the predilection for rounded linear movement and tended to move more angularly like his mother (Illustration 1b). At that time, Charlie began to relate to his mother in a curt, flippant manner, which was similar to her own mode of relating. At the end of adolescence, both Glenda and Charlie developed longer intervals between reversals than they had before. The question arises whether this change is an expression of a greater constancy in relating.

In Nancy's case, angular, linear movements, alternating between high and low amplitudes, characterized her neonatal creeping. We find a striking similarity to that type of shape-flow-design in her current record (see Illustration 1). Surveying this and other recent notations, we discover that they lack the variability and the spread between reversals that we perceive in the records of Glenda and Charlie. Geometric figures, mostly small triangles, and some long, narrow forms, indented at the top, repeat themselves in a crowded manner; they have the quality of tools or machines. Since infancy, Nancy looked more like an animated marionette than a baby. Until late adolescence, she often gave the impression of functioning mechanically. Today, there is a greater animation in Nancy, and her use of effort and shaping make her appear more like one of her sisters. Yet, the style of her relatedness has not changed. Not only the abundance of "cog-wheel" rhythms, but also the frequent reproduction of almost identical, sharp geometric figures distinguishes Nancy's shape-flow-design from that of other subjects. It remains to be seen whether infants with similar shape-flow characteristics will prove to be candidates for mechanical object-relations.

It is very likely that rhythms of shape-flow-design are representative of specific modes of relating[7]), while the intrinsic attributes of these rhythms pinpoint the traits which make a person appear remote, likeable, annoying, extroverted or introverted.

Rhythms of tension-flow and shape-flow-design are ubiquitous. They are noted in all movement serving survival through need-satisfaction and through appeals for nurturance. As development progresses, they gradually come under the service of the ego and undergo changes, not only in accordance with maturation, but even more so in conformance to environmental models. The ego not only is instrumental in the taming of drives and their expres-

---

[7])
Werner (1948) and Ferrari (1969, personal communication) attempted to correlate design with feelings, but without an available classification of modes of object- and self-directedness and their qualities they could not succeed in ordering their information in a meaningful way. Gottschalk (1968) has begun to classify relatedness from verbal samples of behavior. We are looking to his further studies, hoping that they will enable us to classify shape-flow-design rhythms.

sion, but also in the acculturation of corresponding modes of relatedness. While we are not yet able to classify rhythms of shape-flow-design, we are inclined to believe that the ratio of varying rhythmic units is subject to change through development. They may, as is likely in Nancy's case, remain unaltered when the ego has not succeeded in making the originally preferred forms of relating subservient to social aims.

CHAPTER 5

IDENTIFICATION OF SPECIFIC MOTOR RHYTHMS AS
EXPRESSIVE OF SPECIFIC DRIVES SUCH AS ORAL,
ANAL, PHALLIC AND OTHERS

Section I

Sources of Criticism and Differences in Definition

Critics of our system of notation and interpretation
have questioned the terms we use to denote specific tension-flow rhythms. It has been suggested that the rhythms we notate and score should not be classified in
accordance with the nomenclature "reserved" for drive
components, because, in doing so, we run the risk of im-
plying that motor rhythms are identical with drives. In
psychoanalytic literature, however, we speak of "oral
drives" and "oral characters" without equating them. We
also speak of "anal zones" without equating them with anal
wishes or anal traits. Nevertheless, we have applied
quotation marks, or have spoken of "types" of rhythms, to
help readers distinguish between an "oral" rhythm (that
is, an oral type of rhythm) and an oral drive. This is
especially useful when we speak of "libidinal" (libidinal-
type) and "sadistic" (sadistic-type) rhythms. Despite
these safeguards, there still remains the implication, not
of sameness, but of correlation. This is justified, for
such a correlation does exist. Moreover, our classification is useful to the clinician because it avoids non-
specific categorization.

Non-analytic critics reproach us for introducing
Freudian terms into the classification of movement. Some
would like movement to be viewed on its own terms, without
interpretation; others would like interpretations to be
more in keeping with terminology understood by laymen. We
have introduced movement terms for the classification of
rhythms so that those who study movement exclusively will
be able to use them. For "oral" rhythms we speak of "sucking" and "biting" or "snapping-type" rhythms; for "anal"
rhythms we use the terms "twisting" and "straining"; for
"urethral" rhythms we speak of "running" and "run-stop-go"
types; for "inner-genital" rhythms we use the terms "undulating" and "swaying"; and for "phallic" rhythms we
speak of "jumping" and "leaping". It is immediately appar-

ent that this classification is in no way as accurate as the one derived from psychoanalytic terminology. However, it is descriptive enough to give a fair impression of the movement involved.

Another difficulty encountered in the naming of tension patterns arises from the multiple use of the term "tension". Psychoanalysis, for instance, has usurped this word to connote a damming up of instinctual drives calling for release. Metaphors, derived from free- and bound-flow, are applied to the construct of psychic energy. Reich (1927) measured the degree of defensiveness (psychic armor) by the rigidity of patients' muscles. Jacobson (1964) measured the intensity of tension as contrasted with relaxation. To him, as to Reich and his followers, tension meant a high degree of boundness and relaxation meant an extreme limpness (which would make the jaw drop).

To us, tension reflects the elastic qualities of living tissue. It ranges from boundness to release of tension in free flow. Limpness and inertia are indications of a loss of elasticity. Our notations pertain to the changes in tension during movement; we do not notate the state of muscles at rest, commonly called tonus. Rather, we follow Lamb and Turner (1969) who record variations in the quality of a motion factor instead of the persistence of a quality (North, 1972). The basic polarities of movement, a tightening in bound flow and a release in free flow, are encompassed by our use of the term "tension". These polarities represent bridges between soma and psyche, serving as passage-ways for the transformation of neural impulses and inhibitions into the psychic polarities of feeling safe or feeling anxious (Sandler et al, 1969).

For Laban (1960), tension was included in his concept of efforts. This concept encompassed not only actions related to space, gravity and time, but also to the "flow of effort". When, with Lamb's help, Irma Bartenieff and I discovered that efforts are not available at birth, I asked myself what was flowing in the movements of the newborn. It seemed to me that Laban's own definitions of free and bound flow, as resulting from an interplay between antagonistic and agonistic muscles, implied that his "flow of effort" was based on the elasticity of motile tissue. No doubt, all movement patterns must proceed in a flow which either releases or inhibits them, but it is not useful to single out the "flow of effort" as if flow were the medium of efforts alone.

Giving the appellation "flow of tension" to Laban's "flow of effort" was one of the ways in which we sub-

divided the global term "effort" into its components.
For Laban, efforts encompassed a great many clearly differentiated psychological characteristics. He referred
to efforts as "impulses", but also as "drives". In the
then accepted meaning of the term "Trieb", Laban's concept
was not different from Freud's "Trieb" (meaning an instinctual drive). In addition, efforts could be used for
coping with the environment and for self-protection (i.e.,
as defenses). As "positive" or "fighting" effort elements, they served the fulfillment of active, aggressive
aims; as "negative" or "indulging" effort elements, they
served the fulfillment of passive, libidinal aims (Kestenberg and Marcus, 1977). Combinations of two efforts
signified such affective attitudes as remoteness or
stability. Combinations of three efforts were called
"basic" or "full" efforts, exemplified in a punch or a flic
For our purposes, we divided Laban's efforts into tension-
flow (serving the expression of needs, affects and drives),
precursors of efforts (used for defenses), and effort
proper (operative in the struggle of the individual with
the forces of external reality).

Section II

Tension-Flow Rhythms as the Apparatus For Need- and Drive-Satisfaction

Tension-flow rhythms are part of our congenital physic
equipment which is, at first, independent of the psyche.
Hypothalamic centers regulate rhythmicity of organs, zones
and systems. There is a correlation between secretory and
motor rhythms, as seen for instance in the interrelation of
adrenaline secretion and vigorous motor discharge or in
the chain-reaction of prolactin-secretion, milk production
and its ejection through contractions of mammary ducts. No
one doubts that the psyche is influenced by and exerts an
influence over these rhythmic somatic processes. Both the
involuntary and the voluntary muscle systems are subject to
the mutual influence of soma and psyche. A basic conformity between motor rhythms of striate (voluntary) and non-
striate (involuntary) muscles is exemplified in the interaction between eating and gastric contractions.

Although the rhythmic functions of the neonate are
not fully developed, they are already subject to the laws
of periodicity that connect specific rhythms to specific
systems, organs and functions. Very likely, an oral type

rhythm is used not only in the oral zone, but in the whole alimentary system, with the inclusion of all functionally related body parts. For instance, the sucking rhythm is very similar to certain peristaltic rhythms. The distal ends of the upper extremities, which at first serve as feeding utensils, are frequently engaged in tension-flow rhythms which we classify as "oral". Our experience shows that oral type rhythms are used in all parts of the body, but are most frequent in the perioral zone and in finger play. There seems to be a readiness in all body parts to assist in the functioning of alimentation and other fundamental systems, when needed. In addition, there are frequent rehearsals in play actions which keep all mechanisms of survival fit for use at all times.

In interaction with the environment, the infantile rhythms become increasingly better differentiated. The mother serves as a mediator between the baby and the extrauterine influences to which he must adapt. She helps regularize rhythms and encourages the child to choose these appropriately for specific functions. The neonate has at his disposal all rhythm variations which he will use in his life time. However, they are not as differentiated as they will become through maturation, practice in the appropriate zone and interaction with an organizing caretaker. Within this framework (that is, when an organ, or zone, and an object, along with their functions and discharge modes, become the central foci for the obtainment of need satisfaction), needs begin to be represented by wishes, and thus a bridge between soma and psyche is born.

Freud (1915) postulated that drives (the psychic representatives of needs) are characterized by their source in a bodily zone, their discharge process (which he called impetus), their aim and the object to which they are directed. Taking as an example the oral drive, its source is the snout-zone; its typical discharge proceeds through the use of "oral" sucking tension-flow-rhythms; its aim is to obtain satisfaction for incorporative needs and its object is the nipple or the baby's finger. Hunger contractions trigger the stimulation of the oral cavity to which the baby responds by mobilizing spontaneous rooting. Mouthing and sucking motions ensue. Autoerotic, non-nutritive sucking gives the baby more opportunity to practice moving in "oral" tension-flow-rhythms after hunger has been stilled. This play-practice, which substitutes for hunger-relieving motions, is not only used for the sake of rehearsal and preparation for proper muscle-functioning during the next meal, but also for the stimulation of salivary secretion in anticipation of it. Through this practice the baby begins to differentiate his finger (that is felt and feels) from the nipple (that is felt but does not feel). Furthermore, through this practice, a division is made between the total incorporation of the undifferentiated nipple-milk object and the incomplete and transitory incorporation of object, hand or finger.

We can easily see that the tension-flow apparatus is responsible for the impetus (discharge mode) which makes incorporation possible. The moving in and out of the nipple or finger are accomplished with the equipment we have named "shape-flow-design".

The successive growing and shrinking of lips, which protrude to seize and retract during swallowing, utilize the apparatus we have called "shape-flow" (see pp. 77-82). The shape of the mouth in seizing, holding of the object and releasing it provides the experience which will enable the baby to identify the object by its shape.

It would be tempting to pursue the analysis of each drive in this manner. Suffice it to say that the more delayed the maturation of an organ system, the more complex its functioning and the more mental preparation is needed to make it work in a faultless way. In addition, there are several stages of maturation, with the newer stages requiring an increasingly more precise psychic control system. For instance, in the transition from sucking to biting and to chewing of solids, the oral zone is extended by the activation of jaws and an increased versatility of the tongue allows for a greater interaction between various parts of the oral cavity. The aim of the drive is still incorporation, but the now prominent aggressive aspect of destroying the object before swallowing changes its nature. The discharge form becomes modified, with "oral-sadistic" rhythms predominating. The nature of pleasure changes as well, when pain becomes associated with the new function (Kestenberg, 1971, 1975). The separation between the feeding caretaker and food as separate objects becomes more distinct; food becomes a bridge to the mother rather than part of her. Still more complicated is the later transition from a feeling that feces and urine are being eliminated to a conscious control over their functioning.

Needless to say, in each new step towards drive differentiation there is a greater participation by the ego. Rhythms of tension-flow which were available to the newborn are becoming successively more subject to ego-control when a drive-zone, its impetus, aim and object become integrated into a smoothly operating functional system. As a result, precursors of defenses and primitive modes of adaptation lose their previous impact and become replaced by advanced mental mechanisms. For

instance, biting as a primitive response to pain gives
way to isolation while at the same time (or later?) a
greater precision in moving food to the mouth becomes
the preamble to self-feeding. Accordingly, the separation from the object increases and reaching the object
and interaction with the caretaker are transacted in
space. The movement patterns which become distinct in
conjunction with psychic differentiation in the second
half of the first year are:

> Tension-Flow Attributes (with the holding of even
> levels of tension becoming more frequent and more
> prolonged);

> Precursors of Effort and their mature forms (with
> channeling of spatial pathways and a direct
> approach to space becoming more distinct);

> Shape-Flow-Design (with an increase in linear
> pathways which counteract meandering);

> Shape-Flow Dimensions and directions in space
> (with the former initiating reaching across the
> body through narrowing);

> Shaping of Space in Planes (with enclosing in the
> horizontal - the feeding plane - limiting the
> play-space of the high-chair infant and his mother).

The foregoing example of development in the oral
phase will suffice here to highlight the rationale of our
method: we classify motor patterns in movement terms and
in correspondence to the somatic and mental functions
they are related to. More will be said about transitions
from earlier to more advanced patterns and about the
affinity between them in Chapter 6. In the meantime, I
shall turn my attention to the methods we used to arrive
at the classification of tension-flow rhythms.

Section III

Methods Used to Classify Tension-Flow-Rhythms

Among the many ways we used to classify tension-flow
rhythms I shall discuss here the five which yielded the
best results. None of them has been as yet statistically

verified.[8]) We use insight derived from them to check and re-check hypotheses in the same manner as new insights are validated in psychoanalysis.

The following methods will be discussed below:

1. Direct observation and notation of infants' movements.
2. Observation and notation during psychoanalytic sessions.
3. Experimentation with a myograph.
4. Longitudinal studies.
5. Comparison of movement profiles with psychoanalytic assessments.

1. Infant Observation and Notation of Infant Movements.

We notated tension-flow changes in a given zone in which a need-satisfying activity took place, as for instance during sucking or biting. From these notations we could extrapolate the rhythms most advantageous for particular forms of gratification. We noted that performance with deviant rhythms led to a disturbance of function. For example, the use of "phallic" rhythms during nutritive sucking resulted in gulping and choking.

We notated tension-changes during snapping and biting; we noted movements of the anal sphincter, which occurred during wiping or raising of the legs. We notated tension changes before and during defecation and urination, and during masturbatory activities.

Notating during successive developmental phases, we observed that at the peak of each developmental phase certain rhythms were used more often than others. A variety of rhythms could be used for defecation and urination, depending on the nature of the activity. There was more uniformity in inner-genital and phallic rhythms. Swaying, intense inner-genital rhythms were rare, especially in children.

2. Psychoanalytic Sessions.

At times it was possible to notate movement patterns during psychoanalytic sessions. Children particularly

---

8) Using a system devised by Elaine and David Schnee, we are presently in the process of converting symbols into numbers. This will allow for statistical computerization of our data.

were very interested in the method and repeatedly asked me to use it. In one instance a nine year-old boy told me that he used many ways to rub his upper lip while sucking. He asked me to guess (analyze) the meaning of each rubbing mode, and he demonstrated them very willingly. When I told him in simple words what each rubbing style suggested to me, he agreed that he had fantasies of that kind, but had not connected them with what he did with his finger. For example, the use of an "oral" rhythm suggested a wish to suck from the breast, an "anal" rhythm a wish to be wiped and a "phallic" rhythm a wish to make his penis jump up. Such experiences showed me that autoerotic activity in one zone may, but may not, be connected with corresponding drives. These displacements from one part of the body to another are recognized in verbalizations of patients, but the analysis of tension-flow rhythms in special parts of the body can help recognize the route of displacement with greater precision.

Notating tension-flow changes in movements of adult patients during silences or during times of repetitious meandering, can also help link unexpressed ideational content with the prevalent motor discharge form. When the resistance is overcome, the latent wish that influenced the choice of a particular rhythm emerges from obscurity. An accurate correlation between drives and rhythms can be obtained when notation of tension-flow rhythms is undertaken at a time when a clearly identifiable sensation or fantasy betrays its drive-specific origin. For instance, while telling me about her emerging vaginal sensations, a patient rubbed her hand in an inner-genital rhythm. Illustrating with gestures how a car stopped ahead of hers on the road, a patient, who pictured crashing into the vehicle, used predominantly "phallic-sadistic" leaping rhythms.

3. Myograph Experiments.

We attached the electrodes of a myograph to the biceps of two different subjects in successive experiments. After a short interval, the subjects were asked to think of certain activities which could easily be connected with specific needs. In both subjects, the curves seen on the oscillograph changed with the entrance of new thoughts. Moreover, the rise and fall of the curves closely resembled the rhythmic units we have notated free-hand when we were able to correlate ideational content with movement. For instance, a thought of sucking promptly evoked curves identical with our "oral" rhythms. Thoughts of defecation evoked curves very similar to those we have classified as "anal-sadistic". These experiments suggested a correlation between specific drive-dependent thoughts and specific muscular rhythmic discharge forms.

4. <u>Longitudinal Studies</u>.

The longitudinal study of our three subjects was undertaken to develop a means of notation which would be representative of movement patterns, and to develop an approach to the interpretation of these patterns as they reveal psychic functioning. In the childhood of these subjects, we have had to rely on non-systematized descriptions of their movements contained in their earlier records. In addition, we have been able to reconstruct some data from memory. As the system of notation progressed, the description of movement became more precise as well. Since 1965, when the children were twelve years old, I have been able to obtain profiles of each of them on a yearly basis. At times, Irma Bartenieff accompanied me, notated and also constructed profiles. Discussing our respective profiles allowed us to compare our respective notations and to come to a better understanding of our agreements and our differences. This type of collaboration was especially fruitful since we had shared our experiences in observing newborn babies in the Long Island Jewish Hospital.

Since 1972, I have been able to observe children from earliest infancy to three-to-four years of age in the Center for Parents and Children, sponsored by Child Development Research. In doing so, I have come to the conclusion that some of the data derived from the longitudinal study of Charlie, Glenda and Nancy, even though imprecise and incomplete, have stood the test of time. A clear correlation between rhythms of tension flow and clinical data on which we base our assessment of drive could be seen in many examples, out of which I shall single out four.

At the time Glenda's brother was born, an increase in what we now call "oral-sadistic" rhythms coincided with her openly expressed oral-sadistic wishes towards him. In adolescence, when Charlie's profile showed an influx of "biting" ("oral-sadistic") rhythms, he used a great many phrases in which he playfully referred to biting.

Charlie insisted that his mother stay with him in the bathroom long after he was able to toilet himself. His interest in his penis, to which he referred to as "boy", was pronounced, but he treated it as if it were his child. At that time, rhythms, retrospectively identified as "inner-genital", contributed to Charlie's low-key and gradual manner of mobilizing himself. During adolescence, Glenda's appearance was progressively feminized. At that time and even more so during her pregnancy, her record indicated a considerable increase of "inner-genital" rhythms.

In the beginning of the study, I could account only for a few rhythms which stood out in the children's behavior. When members of the movement-study-group began to systematically score records of notation, they encountered regularly recurring rhythmic units which had not been classified as pure and could not be easily interpreted as mixed rhythms. These rhythms were eventually identified as "urethral" and "inner-genital". The existence of the former could not be established until we compared data from my longitudinal study with those obtained from neonates and toddlers and from self-observation and notations of rhythms of various group members. Witnessing the changes that occurred in the newborn rhythm-repertoire within a few days after birth, we began to distinguish between the neonatal, pure "inner-genital" rhythms and mixtures of "oral", "urethral" and "anal" rhythms. In our current work with infants and toddlers, A. Buelte and myself can assess a toddler's readiness for toilet training from the degree to which "anal-sadistic" and later "urethral-sadistic" rhythms are differentiated and from the frequency with which the child uses them. We regularly note the occurrence of "inner-genital" rhythms in maternal behavior of two-and three-year-old children. However, despite our agreement about the classification of rhythms, we still encounter records or passages which present difficulties in scoring. Further work may uncover rhythms not yet classified.

5. <u>Comparing clinical assessments with movement profiles (See appendix).</u>

Since the movement profile (MP) is structured in diagrams, representing the ratio of attributes rather than their single values, it is possible to compare it with data from a dynamic psychological assessment (Freud, A., 1965). When such comparisons were made in the Hampstead Clinic in London and in the Child Development Center in New York (Dr. Neubauer, Director), we found an excellent agreement between the two methods of assessment. The interpretation that the individual's rhythm constellation, as seen on the profile, corresponds closely to his drive constellation, has been confirmed in a number of cases in which neither the history nor the diagnosis, made by the staff, was known to the notators and interpreters of the MP. It is our impression that the overt contents of fantasies or wishes, expressed verbally, are not as reliable indicators of the underlying drives as are the movement patterns which we classify as rhythms of tension-flow.

In analyzing verbal productions, we may find it difficult to distinguish between the drive impetus, its aim

and its object. In addition, we have to consider the
defensive aspects of what has been said without losing
track of the variety of affects expressed and the manner
of coping with external problems, all present at the same
time. Investigators who use descriptive reports of movement encounter the same difficulty. One phrase of a
movement or one gesture may contain, in a more or less
distinctive way, all patterns of movement the individual
is capable of using. By notating patterns rather than
describing the functional aspect of movement, we were
able to isolate discharge modes which are suitable for
specific drive discharge. We discovered the characteristics of rhythms which revealed drive aims in broader
terms of "libidinal" and "sadistic". We learned that
there was an affinity between tension-flow and shape-
flow, indicative of the intrinsic connection between the
drive-impetus and the drive-object. However, we do not
yet have a model suitable for the establishment of a
classification of rhythms which would isolate specific
modes of relating, as for instance the specific approach-
withdrawal rhythm of the oral or the anal child.

We have not yet invented ways of writing continuous
shape-flow changes, and the notation of shape-flow-design
is probably insufficient to cover the data needed to
assess the forms relationships take in early development.
We anticipate that each tension-flow rhythm is coordinate
with only a limited number of shape-flow and shape-flow-
design rhythms to allow for the optimal interaction with
an object, in the service of drive satisfaction which
guarantees survival.

In summary, we note that we have used a number of
methods to identify and classify tension-flow rhythms.
We have yet to find means of identifying shape-flow and
shape-flow-design rhythms so that we can appraise an individual's drive constellation on the basis of his interaction with objects.

---

9) The difficulty arises from our inability to represent
three-dimensional patterns within the two dimensions
of the paper on which we notate, and from the fact
that our consecutive notation of shape-flow-design
changes suffers from the failure to reproduce simultaneous changes in various parts of the body. For in
stance, an arm may reach out while the other comes
close to the body. We can only roughly estimate
whether there is more or less movement towards or awa
from the body.

CHAPTER 6

TRANSITIONS BETWEEN DRIVE-
AND EGO-DEPENDENT MOTILITY

Tension- and shape-flow rhythms can be noted in all movement. Super-imposed on these rhythms are more advanced movement patterns, namely, effort and shaping of space. Although they mature later, they evolve from attributes of body-tension and body-shape respectively. They are measures of ego-development, as they are used by the ego to achieve its aims. Through their influence on tension-flow and shape-flow they can modify and deflect drive expressions and subordinate them to ego interests and goals.

In posing the question about the transition of drive- to ego-dependent motility, we didn't, at first, distinguish between rhythms and attributes. Our studies indicate that one can predict preferences for certain effort elements not from rhythms, but rather from early preferences for certain attributes of tension-flow, which regulate rhythms. For instance, the frequency of Glenda' accelerations could be predicted from the fact that she had a tendency to change tension abruptly, an important feature of the phallic rhythms.

The developmental line from tension-flow attributes to efforts suggests that specific affects, experienced in infancy, play a role in the choice of later modes of adaptation to external reality. For instance, an abrupt, impulsive baby with a low capacity to delay gratification will be inclined to grow into an impatient, hurried adult who tends to beat time by acceleration.

In the early stages of this study, we did not distinguish between tension-flow and shape-flow rhythms. With the extension of our knowledge into the realm of shape-flow and shaping, we opened up an inquiry into the developmental line from early to later forms of relating through movement. An example of a transition from a specific preference for a shape-flow attribute to the later-developing preference for a shaping element can be drawn from the case of Charlie. He tended to widen as an infant, and later developed a predilection for moving sideways (laterally) and for spreading in space. Such a developmental correspondence can be close in all patterns of shape. For instance, an early tendency to move towards the body in linear pathways and to narrow symmetrically and asymmetrically may forebode a preference for moving across the body and for enclosing small segments of space. This can be interpreted to mean that a clear-cut, narcissistic, clinging (through narrowing) form of early relating will presage the development of closed, circumscribed (across the body) and possessive (enclosing) traits in relation to objects.

Records of profiles taken in successive developmental phases indicate that what appears to be a forerunner of an advanced pattern sometimes becomes incorporated into the advanced pattern and ceases to exist independently of it. At other times, we see that a preferential early pattern persists with or without a corresponding preference for its more mature counterpart. An example of the former is the disappearance of widening in Charlie's adolescence and a persistent preference for moving sideways and spreading (see his latest profile in the appendix, p.130). Examples of the latter, as seen in Glenda's profile, are the persistence of preferences for all three: abruptness, suddenness and acceleration, and for lengthening without an emphasis on moving upward.

In this chapter, I will discuss the transitions from tension-flow to efforts and from shape-flow to shaping. I will include a section on affinity between patterns in order to pursue the developmental line from the affinity between tension- and shape-flow to the matching of effort and shaping elements. This aspect of the study opens up the vista for a better understanding of transitions from early modes of harmony or clashing to later conflict-free or conflict-laden functioning. The last section of this chapter will cover the developmental line from the exclusive use of gestures to the employment of gesture-posture sequences (Lamb, 1969). A clinical example of this type of transition is the derivation of the superego's observing function from the ego's capacity for undivided attention, turned inward. This line of research is beginning to probe the significance of movement patterns in the transition from ego- to superego-controlled behavior.

All patterns available to the newborn remain in the adult's movement repertoire. However, with progressive development, the ego gains at least partial control over the early patterns and becomes instrumental in reducing their frequency and in subordinating their aims to those of advanced motion factors. In this process, tension- and shape-flow attributes become partially incorporated into efforts and shaping, respectively. The transition from a flow attribute to an effort or shaping element proceeds along the lines of specific affinities between patterns.

There is insufficient material in this pilot study to document each proposition regarding the transitions from early to later development of motility. However, because they all constitute vital ingredients of the outcome of this study and have become incentives for specific research, many of them will be taken up in the following sections. By necessity, there will be a certain amount of overlapping with previous chapters, with some topics covered in detail and others mentioned only in passing.

Section I

From Tension-Flow Attributes to Precursors of Effort and Efforts

(From drive- and affect-regulation to the control of learning, of defenses and of coping behavior)

To preface this section I shall review the definitions of terms and the suggested correlation between a motion pattern and its psychic representation.

Rhythms of tension-flow consist of rhythmic units which repeat themselves in regular and irregular intervals. Each unit has qualities which vary and those which are obligatory. The latter must be present for a rhythmic unit to be classified as a pure rhythm. Mixed rhythms can be recognized by the traces of the qualities which characterize the component rhythms. The qualities of tension-flow which regulate rhythms are: free or bound flow, even or readjusting levels of tension, high or low intensity, and abrupt or gradual rate of change in progression from free to bound flow and vice versa. For instance, a "phallic" rhythm must be abrupt, but its intensity changes. Flow regulation controls the choice of rhythmic units and their sequence.

Rhythms of tension-flow can be correlated with specific drive-discharge modes (Freud's impetus) which are derived from organ modes and become a source for the modalities of wishing. For instance, "oral" rhythms, which are derived from oral sucking, are the motor expressions of oral drives which probably give rise to hallucinatory types of wishing to incorporate.

Tension-flow attributes contribute their share to a class of affects in which danger and safety are a consideration, with bound flow used when feeling cautious and free flow used when feeling carefree. Shades of affect vary depending on the combinations of tension-flow attributes and other motor patterns. As a result, one tension-flow attribute can be correlated with a variety of feelings. For instance, high intensity of tension levels is used in anxiety attacks, in temper and in exuberance. The fact that flow-regulation controls rhythms of tension-flow via the selection of tension-flow attributes suggests the following line of thought: Affect regulation is the intermediate step in the control of drives which cannot be dealt with directly. Flow regulation is intrinsic to tension-flow rhythms. At the same time, it is an intrinsic component of the patterns we call precursors of effort.

Precursors of effort make use of a tension-flow attribute to pursue the aims of effort during learning. For instance, in learning how to reach, a child will attempt to keep his tension level even in order to channel his movement in space. "Channeling" is a precursor of direct effort elements. Once reaching has become automatized, the child will use an appropriate effort element; he will move directly to the object. Precursors of effort are the motor components of defenses; for instance, "channeling" is used in isolation and "vehemence" in identification with the aggressor.

Efforts are motion elements used in the adaptation to space, gravity and time. They are the motor components of the ego's adaptation to external reality. For instance, acceleration is an important aspect of an individual's adaptation to the realities of time. An example of the transition from tension-flow regulation to precursors of effort and effort is the developmental line from using even flow to its incorporation in channeling and its integration into directness.

The use of even levels of tension-flow is typical for people whom we call "unruffled" or even-tempered. Since this implies a rather infrequent use of flow fluctuations, it is expected that the same people are not spontaneous and will not be subject to frequent affect reversal. The preference for even tension levels can be seen in some newborns who are capable of remaining calm or of retaining the same level of excitation for shorter or longer periods of time. When such an unruffled infant moves his arm and brings his hand close to his mouth, he tends not to derail from his aim. When he begins to reach for objects, he can make use of this tension-flow attribute to channel the pathways in space which lead to the objects he

seeks. Calmness and steadiness become part of
his native equipment which he will use automatically to pay focussed attention. He will approach
space directly and this quality will stand him in
good stead when he will be required to concentrate.

The tension-flow apparatus has at its disposal a
primitive protective mechanism (Stern, 1951). The binding of tension-flow reduces mobility or stops it altogether, forming the basis for immobilization through
fright. The freeing of tension-flow initiates activity,
forming the basis of mobilization for flight. Another
primitive protective mechanism is deanimation, which,
through the loss of elasticity, produces neutral flow.
Clinically, neutral flow appears in literary descriptions
in such terms as wooden, waxen, like stone, like molasses,
watery, slippery, like a rag doll, etc.

Nancy's use of the protective mechanism of
bound flow was excessive, a tendency which diminished as time passed by. She alternated this
mechanism with the use and abuse of neutral flow.
Even though this diminished considerably, there is
still evidence that Nancy becomes inert or limp
more often than the average person. Charlie, who,
as an infant, withdrew into "dazes" also uses a
good deal of neutral flow today but much less so
and more selectively than Nancy. Glenda still
tends to mobilize herself through free flow, which
facilitates displacement.

It is difficult to say which psychic agency regulates
the primitive protective mechanisms of mobilization
through release into free flow, immobilization through
binding and deanimation through neutral flow. We are
dealing here with a borderland between the id and the
body-ego which does not permit clear differentiation
(Kestenberg, 1953). Gradually, the ego takes over limited control over these mechanisms. Bound flow can be
instituted at will, but release into free flow is more
difficult to obtain without special training. Voluntary
activation of neutral flow is possible. However, it requires a transitory suspension of the affective components of higher ego-functioning.

Regulation of tension-flow attributes is intrinsic
to the later-developing affect control. One can divide
the tension-flow attributes into those which occur more
often in frustration and those which indicate relief
and achievement of satisfaction. The trio of high intensity of tension, developed abruptly and held on an
even level is a combination of three tension-flow attributes, each of which serves as an expression of and a
response to frustration. Conversely, the trio of low

intensity, developed gradually with adjustments of tensions levels, is a combination which is a frequent expression of and response to gratification.

High intensity, abruptness and holding tension on an even level in bound flow come to the fore separately or together in negative affects such as temper, impulsivity, stubbornness and anxiety. Low intensity, graduality and adjustment of tension-level in free flow are generally marks of positive affects, such as pleasantness, patience, playfulness and ease. It is immediately apparent that the former represent more active and the latter more passive strivings (Kestenberg and Marcus, 1977). It is likely that changes from one attribute to another or variations of sets of tension attributes underlie such early defenses as turning from passivity to activity and vice versa, reversals of affect, flattening of affect and distractibility through displacement, and the earliest forms of identifications with the aggressor and reaction formations.

While reports on attributes of tension-flow are incomplete for the early stages of the three subjects, some data are available. It is known, for instance, that already in infancy, Glenda's tendency towards abruptness was tempered by tendencies toward graduality (the motor ingredient of affect-reversal from impatience to patience). She has solved the conflict inherent in the opposition of these two trends by distributing them in phrases in which the beginning of a phrase or the transition into another phrase is frequently abrupt and graduality is more frequent in the main action. This suggests that she now uses a successful reaction formation against impatience, but the original impulsivity has to be activated for a brief time just before the defense becomes operative, as seen in doing and undoing.

Charlie's original conflict between activity and passivity was expressed in his simultaneous use of high intensity and graduality. He has ceased to function as intensely as he used to and does not become as excited as formerly. He prefers low intensity which has become the mainstay of his reaction formation against anger. However, derivatives of high intensity can be detected in Charlie's more advanced defense mechanisms and coping patterns. Today, his conflict between activity and passivity still persists, but expresses itself primarily in his veering from his "learned" abruptness to his originally preferred graduality of tension changes.

Nancy still tends to hold her torso immobile, retaining the same high level of tension as a defense, but she changes levels of tension frequently in her mouth and limbs, especially her wrists and ankles. This type of distribution of tension attributes in different body parts evolved from the long periods of immobilization to which Nancy was subjected in her infancy. At that time she had to hold still while she sucked her bottle, but could make small peripheral movements without losing her balance. This type of partial stabilization is both defensive and adaptive.

We note that tension-flow regulation contributes to the formation of defenses against affects. Thus, the reversal from abrupt tension increase to graduality becomes part of a reaction formation against impulsivity. A wavering between two incompatible tension-flow attributes underlies the early forms of doing and undoing.

<u>Precursors of effort</u> can be seen in transitions from <u>tension-flow regulation</u>, through the selection of one or more attributes of tension, to the control of the environment through the use of <u>effort</u>. Whereas flow regulation aims at the control of the body and of affect, effort elements are used to make an impact on the environment. Precursors of effort influence external reality only indirectly. They make use of tension-flow attributes selectively, taking care--so-to-speak--that changes in tension do not interfere with the task at hand. Efforts are concerned almost exclusively with external reality. Through their influence, selection of tension-flow qualities becomes automatized and, yet, there is a greater variability in the choice and sequencing of tension qualities than in precursors of effort. Precursors of effort are frequently rigid because they treat problems posed by external reality in a manner similar to the way flow-regulation deals with internal sources of frustration. They protect the body against danger, but they shift the emphasis from the danger from within to concern with the danger from without.

It has been noted that precursors of effort develop before efforts. In teaching students to recognize precursors of effort, it proved most advantageous to tell them to try hard to do something which they have not yet learned or which is difficult to do. Invariably, like children learning new patterns, the students then pay attention to their own bodies. For a long time, we looked upon precursors of effort as patterns which were typical of learning processes before the learned item could be evoked automatically. When our group began to correlate movement profiles with psychoanalytic assess-

ments and as we became more concerned with the evaluation of activities during which precursors of effort were
used, it became increasingly apparent that precursors of
effort served a great many defense mechanisms.

The observation of the simultaneous use of precursors of efforts in the service of learning and in the
service of defenses brought up the possibility that learning new functions involves the use of defenses. The learner is afraid of injury or of disapproval by the teacher.
Unless he apprehends the new task immediately, he employs
defensive maneuvers to avoid danger while practicing a
skill which he has not yet mastered. In a way, the employment of defenses is used for the learning and re-
learning of methods which keep the individual danger-free.

We do not know all the variables which play a role in
the selection of precursors of effort, which serve learn-
ing-and defense-modes, and in the selection of mature
effort-elements, which are primarily used for coping with
reality, but may also contribute to defensive actions. No
doubt, there is a simple ascendancy from originally preferred tension-flow attributes to preferred precursors
of efforts and to effort elements. A preference may be
preserved in tension-flow as well as incorporated into
precursors of efforts and efforts. In other cases, the
originally preferred tension-flow quality may diminish
absolutely or relatively, becoming absorbed in a preference for a related precursor of effort and/or effort
element.

For a better understanding of the examples that
follow, we list the following patterns as they are devel-
opmentally related:

tension-flow	precursors	efforts	
even flow ⟶	channeling ⟶	directness	(f)
flow adjustment⟶	flexibility ⟶	indirectness	(i)
high intensity⟶	vehemence ⟶ (or straining)	strength	(f)
low intensity⟶	gentleness ⟶	lightness	(i)
abruptness ⟶	suddenness ⟶	acceleration	(f)
graduality ⟶	hesitation ⟶	deceleration	(i)

In this table (f) and (i) indicate the effort elements
Laban classified as "fighting" and "indulging" respectively

In the following examples, PE = precursor of effort
and E = effort.

Glenda continued to use abruptness as well as suddenness (a sequel to abruptness of tension and a PE
of acceleration) and acceleration as her favored patterns. This could be correlated with her impulsivity,
her learning in spurts, her counterphobic behavior,
and her ability to get conflict-free tasks accomplished
on time. Before her pregnancy, she would employ vehemence (a sequel to high intensity of tension and a
PE of strength) and resorted to strength very sparingly. During her pregnancy, the complexity of her PEs
diminished considerably, she reduced her vehement
actions and used more strength than before, combining
it now with directness. (See page 129.) This was
in keeping with the clinical observation that Glenda,
during her pregnancy, became fearful, reduced her
defenses, and was able to function with determination in planning the surroundings for her child.

When Charlie's tendency towards graduality decreased, he increased the frequency with which
hesitation (a sequel to graduality of tension and
the PE of deceleration) as well as suddenness (a
sequel to abruptness and the PE of acceleration)
occurred. In coping with time, Charlie used deceleration and acceleration copiously, but he preferred the former. Delay as a defensive mode of
learning was prominent, but learning by flashes of
insight occurred as well (p.130).   Even though
the frequency of high intensity of tension diminished, he definitely preferred vehemence (a sequel
to high intensity and the PE of strength) over
other PEs. He used it singly in the service of
identification with the aggressor and in combination with channeling and hesitation to uphold and
reinforce a massive repression.

Tempering her abruptness with reversals into
graduality, Nancy at 20 used PEs sparingly and
simply, but she showed a preference for channeling
(a sequel to even flow of tension and a PE of
directness) and for suddenness (a sequel to abruptness and a PE of acceleration). Channeling helped
her to isolate and suddenness aided her counter-
phobic actions. The same patterns characterized
her learning modes. She learned by dividing things
into categories, and in sudden spurts of attention.
Most striking was the absence of gentleness and a
reduced use of vehemence. She seemed to inhibit
too obvious expressions of aggression and had no
recourse to reaction formation against it. In conflict-free functioning, she favored "fighting" over

65

"indulging" elements. Her most frequently used E was acceleration, no doubt a successor to the abrupt jerkiness noticed in her early infancy.

In the foregoing examples I have shown some connections between early preferences for certain tension-flow attributes and related precursors of effort and effort elements, such as:

1) Glenda's abruptness⟶ suddenness⟶acceleration;
2) Charlie's graduality⟶ hesitation⟶ deceleration;
3) Nancy's jerky abruptness⟶suddenness⟶**acceleration**.

However, these developmental lines were by no means the only variables which played a role in the selection of motor patterns, serving learning modes, defense mechanisms and adaptive functions. For instance, Charlie's suddenness and acceleration may be accompanied by abruptness, an attribute which he joyfully embraced when he was stimulated by his mother during his infancy. Nancy's preferences for certain precursors of effort and efforts are not only derived from her early infantile predisposition but are also acquired through her identification with her brothers and her highly intelligent father.

The foregoing data indicate that we may be able to trace preferences for specific ego-controlled patterns, such as efforts, from an early preference for their forerunners in tension-flow. One must also take into account the possibility that an unspecific prevalence of aggressive or erotic components in adulthood may have its antecedents in infancy (Fries and Woolf, 1953; Alpert, Neubauer and Weil, 1956). Tension-flow attributes which are frequently seen in frustration are forerunners of "fighting" efforts and those which are frequently observed in states of satisfaction are forerunners of "indulging efforts" (Laban, 1947). The question arises whether the prevalence of patterns expressing frustration or satisfaction in infancy is a valid indication of a future preference for aggressive or life-sustaining ("erotic") modes of ego functioning. Nancy's case points in this direction. However, even in her, we not only see the environmental reinforcement of what we think was her native inclination to aggress, but we also see the influence of new maturational advances and new opportunities which reduce the impact of this predisposition. This example is typical of the complexity of the problem of the genetic continuity of innate predispositions.

The next question is just as important as the first, and just as difficult to answer. Can one predict the future distribution of aggressive and erotic components from early infantile rhythms of tension-flow rather than from tension-flow attributes? All one can say at this point is that rhythms of tension-flow can be used for the appraisal of sadistic and libidinal discharge forms for which they are suited. Their modes of regulation carry with them distinct qualities which may well presage aggressive and life-sustaining ("erotic") ego traits.

Section II

From Shape-Flow Attributes to the Shaping of Space in Directions and in Planes

(From the regulation of self- and object relatedness to the control of learning, defenses and relating to constant objects)

It is clear from the preceding discussion that the patterns of tension, of precursors of effort and of effort proper are modes and qualities which bear little relationship to objects. Patterns of shape-flow and shaping of space are easily accessible to changes which result from imitation of, identification with, and adjustment to people. They give structure to patterns of tension and effort.

Shape-flow serves intake, output and reactivity to stimuli. It can be used effectively for the transfer of life-sustaining ("erotic") and aggressive impulses from within to without and vice versa. A distinction has to be made between bipolar and unipolar shape-flow and shape-flow design.

Bipolar shape-flow reacts to environmental influences (air, heat, cold, etc.) by symmetrical growing and shrinking. Its attributes are:

1) widening on both sides or narrowing by bringing the two sides closer together;

2) lengthening by stretching upward and downward or shortening by bringing the upper and lower parts of the body closer to the middle; and

3) bulging by stretching the front and back outward or hollowing by bringing the front and back closer together.

Unipolar shape-flow changes the shape of the body

67

in relation to localized stimuli by asymmetrical growing
and shrinking. Its attributes are:

1) widening to one side (laterally) or narrowing on
one side towards the middle (medially);

2) lengthening or shortening towards the head
(cephalad) or towards the bottom (caudad); and

3) bulging or hollowing anteriorly or posteriorly.

Shape-flow design uses the changing shape of the
body (especially limbs) to create a design of the spatial
pathways of centrifugal and centripetal movements. Its
attributes are:

1) looping or linear pathways;

2) low or high amplitudes; and

3) rounded or angular reversals[10)

proceeding from near- through intermediate- to reach-
space or vice versa.

Bipolar (symmetric) and unipolar (asymmetric) shape-
flow and shape-flow-design are available to the neonate,
but they are subject to changes during development.
Feeling big or small, comfortable or uncomfortable, experiencing pleasant and unpleasant sensations in various
parts of the body, which grow towards some and shrink
from other stimuli, and putting one's own body into per-
spective in relation to the space surrounding us, are
all steps in the creation of the body-image. This cannot be accomplished without the simultaneous erection of
the image of an object from whom we differentiate. In
the interplay between the self and others, who are removed from us in space, we begin to extend our dimensional vectors and pathways into spatial directions. Reaching the object in space facilitates the formation of object representations. Through multidimensional shaping
of space, the ego gains access to the expression and
communication of complex relationships to constant objects via the medium of movement.

It is likely that patterns of shape-flow, discernible in the newborn, are part of the innate apparatus
which contains the anlage for patterns of shaping in space
which mature later in life. Preliminary studies indicate
that attributes of symmetrical shape-flow are forerunners

---

10) Formerly called smooth and sharp.

of global, bilateral shaping in planes:

symmetrical shape-flow → global postural shaping in planes

widening ——————→	bilateral	spreading
narrowing ——————→	" "	enclosing
lengthening —————→	" "	ascending
shortening ←—————	" "	descending
bulging ——————→	" "	advancing
hollowing —————→	" "	retreating

Bilateral shaping leads to changes in position through such motions as embracing, jumping and leaping.

Asymmetrical shape-flow may well be a forerunner of shaping in directions, as well as of unilateral shaping in planes:

asymmetrical shape-flow	directional shaping	unilateral shaping in planes
lateral ————→	sideways ————→	spreading
medial ————→	across ————→	enclosing
cephalad ————→	upward ————→	ascending
caudad ————→	downward ————→	descending
anteriorly ————→	forward ————→	advancing
posteriorly ————→	backward ————→	retreating

Unilateral actions are used for responses to stimuli, for localizing points in space, connecting them and pointing to them. They are often used to initiate integrated postural shaping in planes. While bilateral actions cause changes in position from one stable attitude to another, unilateral actions enhance the continuity of motion, that is, mobility.11)

Shape-flow design provides the means of orienting oneself in space, taking one's body as a focal point of departure and return. "Away from me" and "to me" are concepts born from the perception of centripetal and

---

11) I am grateful to Irma Bartenieff for drawing my attention to this distinction.

centrifugal movement. No doubt, growing of body shape is related to going out into space, while shrinking is related to turning back to one's body. This seems to be the basic external pathway for the flow of interactions between the self and objects. Attributes of shape-flow design remain interrelated with attributes of symmetrical and asymmetrical shape-flow. As forerunners of shaping they follow a specific developmental line:

looping→sideways→spreading   linear→across body→enclosing

small——→upward→ascending   large——→downward→descending
amplitude   amplitude

rounded——→forward→advancing   angular→backward→retreating
reversals   reversals

Our knowledge of shape-flow and shaping has come too late to aid in the retrospective reconstruction of more than the bare outlines of these patterns in the early childhood of Glenda, Charlie and Nancy.

References have been made to Charlie's wide, bulging frame. The impression remains that Charlie tended to widen and bulge symmetrically, to shorten asymmetrically and to use rounded reversals in directions. It has been noted that adolescence brought on a change in his permanent body shape and concommittantly he began to lengthen a great deal. At the same time one could note the angularity of his movement. As an infant Charlie preferred moving downward, sideways and forward. His forward movements were styled by his rounded reversals. Today, Charlie prefers moving sideways and across and rarely uses other directions. Under certain circumstances he spreads (in the horizontal plane) and advances (in the sagittal plane) which may be aftermaths of his early widening and bulging, moving sideways and forward. He consistently descends (in the vertical plane), probably as a continuation of his early preference for shortening and moving downward. Despite the paucity of data, Charlie's case can be used to show the epigenesis of shape-flow and shaping patterns. In Glenda the relationships are less clear.

Glenda's initial lengthening and narrowing decreased somewhat in proportion to other qualities of shape-flow and she learned to widen and shorten more as she grew into adolescence and adulthood. However, her original preference for lengthening, both symmetrically and asymmetrically, has remained. Her preferred direction upward is now overshadowed

by sideways motions which correspond to the now
stressed widening. Her favored ascending is now
much less in evidence than descending which she
began to accentuate in adolescence. She still
favors rounding over angular reversals, which makes
her frequent moving backward and retreating less
conspicuous. Falling in love, getting married and
becoming pregnant in quick succession, Glenda has
been subjected to many changes which affected her
body attitude, her body image and her behavior with
people. She identifies more and more with her mother, but she also emulates her husband. Her new
propensity for enclosing (in the horizontal plane)
may have its root in her earlier predilection for
narrowing, but her husband's decided preference for
this pattern very likely plays a role in this change.
It is noticeable that the couple communicates and
plans in a manner new to Glenda. Her ability to
enclose helps her to clarify her plans.

Nancy's tendency to narrow was accompanied by
many linear movements with sharp reversals. Her
development in shaping of space was delayed and
showed little consistency with the antecedents of
shaping.

Some reconstructions could be made in Charlie and
Glenda regarding the developmental lines from shape-flow
to shaping in directions and planes. The known contribution of shape-flow-design to further development was
minimal.

Shape-flow plays a decisive role in the development
of the body-core of images of "self" and "others". Shaping in space becomes an integral part of complex inter-
relationships with objects, not only those perceived outside but also their internalized images. Moving in
directions and in planes is learned in interaction with
people, but it is widely used in their absence. It is
most impressive to see patients on the couch, pointing to
definite locations and moving in planes as if inviting a
response, when they talk about people who are not present, and above all, when speaking of primary and/or
current love objects. In transitions from shape-flow to
moving in directions and planes we see the motor expressions of transitions from the seeking of the drive objects by the id to the forming of relationships by the
ego.

Tension-flow attributes, expressive of feelings derived from body-tensions, are forerunners of precursors
of effort, which serve learning and defenses against
drives. Shape-flow attributes, expressive of feelings

related to the organism's response to the total environment and to isolated stimuli, are forerunners of shaping in directions, which serve learning via the erection of boundaries and defenses against localized objects. Effort elements adaptive motor ego functions have a hierarchically higher control than their precursors and tension-flow attributes. Elements of shaping in planes belong to the sphere of adaptation to objects and, as such, have a higher control function than their predecessors, shaping in directions and shape-flow attributes.

Section III

Affinities, Consonance and Matching; Clashes, Dissonance and Mismatching: Harmony and Conflict

The term "affinity"[12] in movement refers to patterns which are compatible, support each other or fit together.

Attunement between people is based on the sameness or affinity of their patterns. A child feels at one with his mother when they both use the identical tension-flow and shape-flow attributes. Empathy is based on the use of affined but not necessarily identical patterns. A child who, in his upset, uses high intensity of tension feels his mother's empathy when she holds him with an even level of tension. Both are forerunners of "fighting" efforts. An infant who develops tension gradually is pleased when his mother picks him up in a low-tension embrace. Both attributes are forerunners of "indulging" efforts. Attunement turns into understanding when a mother moves in efforts which are related to the infant's tension-flow attributes. For instance, an understanding mother will pick up her jerky and high strung infant with acceleration and strength. She may touch him gently or lightly when she perceives his low tension. In both instances, the maternal ego selects effort elements which are derived from, and affined to, tension-flow attributes which the infant uses at the moment. Similar conditions prevail in the adjustment between mother and infant, which is dependent on the preservation of affinities in shape-flow and shaping. When the infant widens he needs more space which the mother can provide by using an open-shape pattern in shape-flow or shaping.

---

12) The term "affinity" has been extended here beyond its original usage by Laban and Lamb.

Clashes between mother and child are based on a lack of affinity between their patterns. For instance, a mother can meet her child's graduality with abruptness or acceleration. She may respond to his high intensity with low intensity or lightness. Unless mother and child learn from one another and compromise with one another, there will be a clash of temperaments between them. Clashes though, can and do serve a useful function, provided they are not too extensive or incessant. Clashing with his mother, the child learns to differentiate from her and he learns to cope with frustration. When the child uses patterns not appropriate to a given task, his mother's appropriate patterns will clash with his. She teaches him an optimal selection of motion factors for specific functions and, learning from her, he begins to harmonize with her.

In this section, I shall concentrate on affinities and clashes within one individual. While incompatibility with others leads to external conflicts, preferences for the use of incompatible pattern-combinations create a predisposition for internal conflicts. External conflicts become internalized, forming the core of conflicts between id and the ego, and between the ego and the superego.

General and Specific Affinities Within Movement Systems and Between Them.

The two Movement-Systems encompass the Tension-Flow-Effort and the Shape-Flow-Shape entities, the former dealing with internal and external demands and the latter expressive of self-and other-relatedness.

A general affinity in the tension-flow-effort system exists when either "fighting" or "indulging" attributes and elements combine in an action. Thus, affined patterns support either aggressive or life-sustaining goals. In the shape-flow-shaping system all "close-shaped" patterns support the goal of reducing exposure, while "open-shaped" patterns combine to increase exposure.

Affinities within a system are called vertical. Specific vertical affinity combines patterns which are genetically related. The selection of specific, homogeneous vertically affined patterns (such as even flow of tension with channeling or directness, or hollowing with moving backward or retreating) is an ego function. We refer to it as consonance and to corresponding specific clashing as dissonance. (See Affinities Table 1 in Appendix).

73

Affinities between the two systems of movement are called <u>horizontal</u>. They are based on the compatibility of "fighting" and "closed-shaped" or of "indulging" and "open-shaped" patterns, which can be general or specific. An example of a general horizontal affinity is strength combined with retreating. An example of a specific horizontal affinity is lightness with ascending. The selection of specifically related, homogeneous patterns, which are horizontally affined is an ego function. We refer to it as <u>matching</u> of patterns, with dynamic trends in the tension-flow-effort system receiving a specific structure from corresponding forms in the shape-flow-shaping system. A corresponding specific clashing is called <u>mismatching</u>. The matched patterns become dominant in successive developmental phases -- for instance even flow and narrowing in the oral, vehemence and downward movement in the anal or deceleration and advancing in the urethral phases. (Kestenberg et al, 1971; see Affinities Table 2 in Appendix).

Many combinations of patterns, serving definite functions, are composed of clashing attributes and elements. An example is "pressing" in which the "indulging" effort element of deceleration combines with the "fighting" elements of directness and strength. Clashing and harmonizing are intrinsic aspects of the process of variation in movement. The ego not only acts as a mediator between adversary components but it also creates conflict. Forming dissonant or mismatched combinations of patterns need not simply be a failure of the synthetic function of the ego. It can be used to express conflict, as the choreographer does when he creates dissonance by combining strength with ascending and shows the conflict between man's need to conquer and his lofty ideal.

a) <u>Affinities and Clashing in the Tension-Flow--</u>

<u>Precursors of Effort--Effort System</u>

The term "fighting", (referring to contending or positive effort-elements) and its polarity, "indulging", (referring to yielding or negative effort elements) have been introduced by Laban (1947, 1960). Under the former he included bound flow and under the latter free flow. We extended the terms "fighting" and "indulging" to tension-flow-attributes and precursors of effort and we introduced the equation of "fighting" with "aggressive" and "indulging" with "life-sustaining" tendencies. While using these terms generically, we are cognizant of the likelihood that "fighting" tension-flow attributes express aggressive responses to frustration, "fighting" precursors of effort serve to ward off impulses by aggressive means and "fighting" efforts are used in resisting the forces of nature in the process of alloplastic adaptation. Similarly, "indulging" tension-flow attributes are tensional expressions of ease, relief and gratification, "indulging" precursors of effort serve the warding off of impulses by peaceful or loving means; and "indulging" efforts are used in the accommodation to the forces of nature.

In the newborn we can observe affinities and clashes between "fighting" and "indulging" types of tension-flow attributes. With maturation of new and changes in old patterns, there is a progressive increase in the complexity of their interaction.

In Glenda's development we observed that her propensity for abruptness was followed by a preference for acceleration. Today she easily combines the affined "fighting" patterns of abruptness in tension and acceleration in effort. Being impulsive and hurrying are traits which go well together. As an infant Glenda often combined her abruptness with a high intensity of free flow. In one motion there appeared the affined qualities of abruptness and high intensity and the clashing quality of free flow. Impulsivity and a high degree of a spring-like release did not seem compatible with the ease of free flow. Today she still tends to be abrupt, but she often uses low intensity and bound flow with it. One type of affinity and one type of conflict have been replaced by others: abruptness and bound flow are affined, but they both clash with low intensity. Clinical observation has demonstrated an association between these movement patterns and specific qualities of experience. In her early childhood, Glenda's impulsivity would erupt without too much concern on her part. Now she is impulsive and anxious, and is not given to frequent outbursts.

Glenda used to combine abruptness and vehemence with acceleration, which are three different "fighting" qualities. She would restrain her suddenness and would become hesitant when she was faced with a problem of some magnitude. During her pregnancy, she used fewer and less complex defensive motions and she restricted her aggression to a considerable degree. When it did come through, her predilection for suddenness was again quite noticeable. Recently, she has become more direct, and she combines this effort element with deceleration. One of these elements is of the "fighting" and the other of the "indulging" variety. It seems that she has taken over her mother's conflict between a desire to zero in on a problem in a direct manner and a simultaneous wish to delay its resolution.

75

Charlie's early preference for the diverse attributes of high intensity and graduality was
ameliorated when he attuned to his mother and
could become less gradual. Later on, he became
less intense, but his original predisposition for
conflict--seen in his tension-flow--expressed itself in his frequent use of vehemence with hesitation and of strength with deceleration. The conflict between activity and passivity persisted, but
it took on a new form.

In Glenda and Charlie, one could observe the continuation of certain early affinities or clashes between
tension-flow attributes into similar relationships between elements of effort and its precursors. Early
clashes seemed to undergo a series of ameliorations and
reinforcements, some of which resulted in transformations
into affinities and others into a renewal of clashing,
albeit on a higher level. Through identification with
meaningful objects, new conflicts were acquired.

b) Affinities and Clashes in the "Shape-Flow--

Shaping in Directions--Shaping in Planes" System

Shrinking our body-shape as far as we can, we coil
up and roll into a ball, closing off a large area of our
body. Growing as much as we can, we extend, unroll and
open up our body to contact. When we shape space in
directions and in planes, or move our limbs inward and
outward, we either restrict or open up access to the
space around us. The polarities of "closed shape" and
"open shape" pertain to all aspects of shape-flow and
shaping. Shrinking of shape, centripetal movements,
directions pointing to or through the body and the concave forms of shaping in planes are all affined, closed-
shaped patterns. Growing of body shape, centrifugal
movements, directions pointing away from the body and
convex shapes created in space are all affined, open-
shaped patterns. Each of these categories is subdivided
further into three attributes in each type of flow and
three elements in each type of shaping. As a result,
there are a great many affined combinations and a great
many ways of clashing in this system of movement.

Under the heading of open-shapes we can list the
following affined attributes and elements:

Bipolar, symmetrical widening, lengthening
and bulging in the service of intake, which
are associated with feelings of comfort;

Unipolar, asymmetrical movements with which
we react to attractive stimuli;

Agreeable wavy, small and rounded paths of shape-flow-design;

Directing movement sideways, upward and forward to localize objects positioned favorably in relation to us; and

Shaping in planes by spreading, ascending and advancing to invite approach.

Under the heading of closed-shapes we can list the following affined attributes and elements:

Bipolar, symmetrical narrowing, shortening and hollowing, which are associated with feelings of discomfort;

Unipolar, asymmetrical movement with which we re-act to repelling stimuli;

Forbidding, linear, large and angular designs (shape-flow-design);

Directing movement across the body, downward and backward to localize objects positioned unfavorably to us; and

Shaping in Planes by enclosing, descending and re-treating to discourage contact.

When these affinities are not observed, there emerge clashes, only some of which can be discussed here. Growing in inhalation with a simultaneous shrinking away from a source of danger is a weird combination. The same is true of widening and at the same time moving across to the other side of the body. Whenever we move in this clashing way, we experience correlated feelings of conflict between opposite ways of relating to stimuli and objects.

Charlie's widening and bulging were affined open patterns which contrasted with his propensity for shortening. It stands out in my memory that, as a toddler, he used to put his head on his knees in great despair and yet preserved his bulging wide shape. His propensity for directing his movements sideways and forward, as well as downward, not only brought him into a clash with his mother but also represented a conflict of his own. Directing his gaze sideways, forward and down, he not only missed eye-contact with his mother but also gave the impression of someone who had been deflected from his course by a downward pull. Today, Charlie uses bipolar shape-flow sparingly. His preference for small excursions in symmetrical lengthening shows in the frequent craning of his neck or extending of his limbs, as if he wanted to make himself still longer than he is already. His reactivity to stimuli is varied and complex, except that he very rarely widens laterally. Instead, he enjoys moving sideways without widening, but he does narrow when he directs his movement across his body. He moves only infrequently in other directions but has transferred his original preferences for moving forward and downward into frequent advancing and descending. His ability to ascend is increasing, but his open approach to his mother is qualified by his restriction of contact with her to times when he towers over her. No doubt, the conflict expressed in this manner is typical for his age group. Charlie's early affinities and clashes are preserved, but they are distributed differently than they were in his infancy and childhood. In addition, he has increased his repertoire of shaping to include previously shunned patterns. The new distribution shows that Charlie's motor expressions of self-feelings and his way of seeking contact have changed considerably. His early preference for widening has left permanent traces in his predilection to move sideways to contact people. His early preference for bulging and shortening influenced his current mode of relating through advancing and descending, thus opening and closing off contact at the same time. Through his new preference for lengthening, his recent advances in moving across his body and in ascending, Charlie has added new affinities and new clashes to his movement repertoire. Although lengthening facilitates and supports ascending, the latter has a general lack of affinity with moving across and barring access to Charlie's space.

Vertical Affinities and Clashing; Consonance and Dissonance

in Each of the Two Movement Systems

The classification and interpretation of varied areas of harmony and conflict is a painstaking task yet to be accomplished. However, the complexity of affinities and clashing in the two systems of movement (tension-flow-effort and shape-flow-shaping) ceases to be staggering when we consider the complexity of the numerous psychic manifestations of harmony and conflict which are revealed in a small portion of one psychoanalytic session.

Each subsystem can be used for the expression of conflict through the combinations of "indulging" and "fighting" or "open" and "closed" shapes. For instance, abruptness in low intensity can be found in infants who startle easily but do not react intensely to jarring stimuli. This is especially true of immature infants. Caretakers may not hesitate to expose such babies to loud noises because they are considered easy going. When this tendency persists, children, and later adults, may become easily offended without showing it. A tendency to shorten and to bulge gives a confusing picture to the observer. This can happen when an infant begins to defecate during the time he is being filled by nourishment. Later it is seen as the motor expression of the odd combination of low spirits and satiation.

A joining together of strength, deceleration and indirectness of effort produces an action Laban (1947) called "wringing." A useful, adaptive action, it pits the "fighting" effort of strength against two affine indulging effort elements. The depressive patient who wrings his hands in despair is expressing--in an exaggerated form--the latent conflict of the mover who wrings out a wet towel. The wringing action involves an indirect approach and a slowing down to accommodate to the task, while strength is employed in attacking the heavy, soaked towel to reduce its weight through the expulsion of the fluid. In facing the depressed patient who wrings his hands, we recognize the conflict between the aggressive tendency and its counterparts. We can gain more insight from this example when we consider the additional clashing between shaping patterns which may occur during the wringing action. Spreading and advancing may combine with descending, that is, two open shapes with one closed shape. The spreading and advancing will tend to expose the mover and the descending will tend to cover him. This would constitute both an invitation for, and a barring of, contact. Thus we can see in one action the conflict between accommodating--inviting and contending--rejecting tendencies.

Clashes between the "indulging" and "fighting" attributes in the tension-flow subsystem and between the "open-shaped" and "closed-shaped" attributes in the shape-flow subsystem reflect conflicting feelings. Because the ego can assume an only limited control over feelings which are closely related to bodily needs, we assume that such conflicts originate within the psychic agency, called "id". Clashes between "indulging" and "fighting" elements in the "precursor of effort" or "efforts" subsystems, and between the "open-shaped" and "closed-shaped" elements in the "shaping in directions" and the "shaping in planes" subsystems reflect conflicts in the ego. These conflicts operate between incompatible defenses, such as identification with the aggressor and

avoidance, or barring access to the aggressor and enlarging the limits of contact with him at the same time;
they also occur as incompatibilities of two adaptive
functions of the ego, as in directing one's attention
and slowing down, or in the self-and object-oriented
functions of the ego, as in embracing someone and looking
up to another.

In psychoanalysis we refer to conflicts within one
psychic system (id, ego or superego) as intrasystemic
and to those between two psychic systems as intersystemic
(Hartmann, 1939). The latter can be inferred from
clashes between the subsystems "tension-flow" and "precursors of effort" or "effort," and between the subsystems "shape-flow" and the "shaping in directions" or
"shaping in planes". For instance, when an accommodating
"indulging" effort combines with a "fighting" negative
high intensity of tension, we may witness the absurdity
of an angry light touch. A peaceful, considerate form
of adaptation has been invaded by an aggressive impulse.
In the same action we can detect another type of vertical
clashing such as between shortening and ascending. Here
the conflict would pertain to infantile and more advanced
manners of relating. Shortening, born out of a feeling
of smallness or shrinking away from stimuli from above
interferes with ascending which is used to look up to
people or admire them. Taking into consideration both the
tension-effort and the shape-flow-shaping systems, we
would describe the conflict expressed in this example as
one between an angry withdrawal from and a lighthearted
invitation for contact with someone above (e.g. a towering
adult, God).

It is important to distinguish a general vertical
affinity between heterogeneous qualities of motion, sharing a common goal (of "indulging" or "fighting", "opening"
or "closing") from a specific, vertical affinity between
homogeneous qualities, not only sharing a general goal
but also a specific consonance of affects and coping
mechanisms. An example of the former is a harmonious
coexistence of high intensity and acceleration in one
action; an example of the latter is the integration of
high intensity and strength in one action.

In each movement system, all qualities of motion
represented in the profile-diagrams on the same line and
the same side are consonant. An example of consonance in
tension-flow, precursors of effort and effort is the
abruptness, suddenness and acceleration-frequency in
Glenda's profile. An example of dissonance in the shape-
flow-shaping system is Nancy's lengthening which, when
combined with moving in a vertical direction, can only
be used with moving downward. A much more accurate ap-

praisal of vertical consonance and dissonance can be made
by notating phrases of varying motion-factors which occur
in one action. Charlie's unipolar shortening with
descending, Nancy's widening and spreading, Glenda's
sudden decelerations and Charlie's lengthening and descending are examples of consonances and dissonances seen
in notations in symbols. For a complete listing of consonant and dissonant patterns see Glossary.

In this and the foregoing sections I described affinities and clashes in subsystems and between them.
Throughout development we see an increasing trend for the
subsystem clashes to diminish and those between subsystems
to increase. What at first expressed itself as a clash
between two affective components, both interrelated with
drives and evolved from drive regulation, may later manifest itself in a conflict between affects and defenses or
between affects and adaptive mechanisms. What at first
expresses itself as a clash between two opposing self-
feelings may later manifest itself as a conflict between
narcissistic- and object-directed vectors. It seems from
our movement studies that the stronger the ego, the more
it assumes the role of a mediator, with the result that
conflicts--independent of the ego--become transformed into
conflicts between the id and the ego. For instance, a
conflict between sexuality and aggression changes when
aggression is deflected into defensive and coping actions.

The discovery of consonance and dissonance in vertical
affinity enlarges the scope of our understanding of the
relationship between functions evolving on the same developmental line. The peace of mind people seek during work and
in social encounters is based on the consonance between
special feelings and special forms of adaptation and on
the consonance between certain self-feelings and specific
forms of relating. Their dissonance reflects conflicts,
such as can be seen clinically in the plight of the impatient runner who slows down or the mountain-climber who
shrinks away from heights.

Horizontal Affinity and Clashing; Matching and Mismatching,

Balance and Imbalance between the Two Systems of Movement

The many affined combinations between the two systems
are referred to as horizontal. Some are based on general
aspects of coping and relating, such as "indulging" and
"open-shaped" or "fighting" and "closed-shaped" patterns.
Others pertain to specifically related, matched combinations of homogeneous attributes and elements. I cannot
list here the endless combinations of general horizontal
affinities such as can be seen in "open-shaped" advancing
and "indulging" gentleness or in "closed-shape" narrowing

and "fighting" strength. I shall restrict myself to the partial enumeration and discussion of the matching and mismatching of specific, genetically closely related sets of patterns (Kestenberg et al, 1971);

Matching combinations of "fighting" tension-flow attributes and "closed-shaped" bipolar shape-flow attributes:

Bound flow--shrinking
Even flow of tension--narrowing
High intensity of tension--shortening
Abrupt change of tension--hollowing

Matching combinations of "indulging" tension-flow Attributes and "closed-shaped" bipolar shape-flow attributes:

Free flow--growing
Adjustment of tension level--widening
Low intensity of tension level--lengthening
Gradual change of tension level--bulging

Mismatching combinations in these patterns are:

Bound flow--growing
Free flow--shrinking
Even level of tension--widening
Adjustment of tension--narrowing
High intensity--lengthening
Low intensity--shortening
Abrupt change of tension--bulging
Gradual change of tension--hollowing

All movement is composed of sequences of harmonizing and clashing combinations which repeat themselves in regular or irregular intervals. In addition to the generally affined and matching sets of patterns that occur in one action, we note tension-flow changes which are not accompanied by shape-flow change and vice versa. The former lack structure and the latter lack a dynamic impact. When a tension-flow pattern is repeated frequently, but is neither matched nor mismatched by a corresponding shape-flow pattern, and vice versa, there is an imbalance between the two systems. There is a progressive trend from imbalance to balance and from mismatching to matching of specifically related patterns. Since tension-flow reflects bodily needs and shape-flow is more dependent on external influences, the rhythmic repetition of their combinations expresses the congruity or incongruity, the balance or imbalance, between responses to internal and external stimuli. The more affined these combinations the less conflict-prone the individual. The more balance there is between the two systems, the more orderly seems the development.

Charlie, as a baby, most probably abounded in the harmonious matching sets of graduality and bulging and high intensity with shortening; however his widening seemed inappropriate because of the paucity of tension-flow adjustments. Still, among the many clashes Charlie experienced, there was the least clashing between tension-flow and shape-flow attributes. Thus, we need not be surprised to hear at the beginning of his adolescence that "the high degree of affinity between qualities of tension-flow and shape-flow, efforts and shaping indicates that the level of Charlie's object relationships is well integrated with the quality of his ego attitudes" (1967, p. 132, the third paper of this series). Charlie's innate disposition for ego-integration helped him to achieve a high degree of matching between related patterns.

Affinities between patterns, noted at birth, gradually come under the control of the ego. When patterns are _selected_ in accordance with their specific affinity to the homogeneous counterparts in the same system, we assume the existence of a _consonance_ function in the ego; when they are selected in accordance with their specific affinity to their homogeneous counterparts in another system, we speak of a _matching_ function in the ego. This term, created by Lamb (Lamb and Turner, 1969; Ramsden, 1973), retains its usefulness when it is applied to clinical phenomena. For instance, the matching of strength with descending implies that the mover's determination is supported and structured by an appropriate form of showing people what his intentions are. His determination is matched by his expectation of people's responses to it. Strength mismatched with ascending would convey the mover's own disbelief in his power and might induce people to laugh rather than be awed by it.

Matching between effort and shaping elements is a late achievement. It develops gradually and does not become consolidated before latency.

Matching combinations of "indulging" effort and "open-shaped" shaping elements are listed in matching pairs:

Indirectness---spreading
Lightness---ascending
Deceleration---advancing

Transitions

Matching combinations of "__fighting__" effort and "clos
shaped" shaping elements are also listed in matching pair

        Directness---enclosing
        Strength---descending
        Acceleration---retreating

The __mismatched__ combinations of these elements are:

        Indirectness---enclosing
        Directness---spreading
        Lightness---descending
        Strength---ascending
        Deceleration---retreating
        Acceleration---advancing

Children in early latency find it difficult to reconcile their wishes and interests with what is expected
of them. This is expressed in movement through the mismatching of effort and shaping elements. The latency
child practices and accomplishes matching when he acquire
skills by following directions and accepting them as ego-
syntonic. His loves and hates are becoming standardized
on the basis of drive-derivative affectionate relationships with his friends and hostility directed at his
enemies. If he attacks his friends and befriends his
enemies, he betrays his conflicts in the mismatching of
his effort and shaping elements. If a conflict with a
love object is resolved by an inhibition, a multifaceted
ego function such as attention and exploration may be
curtailed, but mismatching of elements of effort and
shaping need not be prominent.

        When Charlie's learning disturbances became con-
        solidated in latency, his capacity to pay attention
        and explore diminished in effectiveness and scope
        while other functions remained intact. He matched
        his effort and shaping well but rarely used direct-
        ness and enclosing which, together, promote atten-
        tiveness to well defined areas of learning, as is
        required of school children. To escape from the
        dreaded school work into fantasy, he adopted a
        pattern which was well matched with his preferred
        spreading, namely indirectness. Fighting off his
        mother and his teacher, in Charlie's case, was a
        matter of self-assertion. I could recognize it
        from Charlie's general behavior and his verbaliza-
        tions and also from the notation of his well matche
        effort-shaping combinations of strength and des-
        cending. In Charlie's record one sees a consistent
        striving to match effort and shape, so that an in-
        crease or decrease in one eventually leads to a
        similar change in the other. There are of course

exceptions to Charlie's superior matching ability
which may be transitory or persistent. In his
latest profile (p.130) his indirectness has decreased, but there is still a persistence of spreading in gestures. A mismatching between directness
and spreading is probably the most noticeable motor
substrate of a conflict which perpetuates Charlie's
learning disability. There is an imbalance when
Charlie descends without strength, trying to appear
determined but not having the stamina to back the
show. As will be discussed in the section on gestures and postures, Charlie's present-day matching
ability is much more pronounced in postural movements than in gestures, but there is still a fair
matching in the latter of lightness and ascending,
deceleration and advancing, and acceleration and
retreating.

A Review of Pattern-Combinations, Expressing Conflict

Conflicts are expressed in movement which does not
follow the rules of affinity. One can detect proneness
to conflict in infants and one can assess its degree
from the frequency with which clashing combinations are
used. Listed below are the areas in which one can detect
predisposition to conflict:

1) In the subsystem clashes of heterogeneous tension-
flow attributes, e. g. graduality and high intensity.

2) In the subsystem clashes between heterogeneous
shape-flow attributes, e.g. lengthening and narrowing.

3) In clashes between subsystems, involving heterogeneous bipolar and unipolar shape-flow and shape-
flow-design attributes, e. g. bipolar widening with
unipolar shortening or lengthening with sharp reversals.

4) In the horizontal clashes of: a) a general nature
between tension-flow and shape-flow attributes, e. g.
tension-flow adjustment with bipolar or unipolar
hollowing and b) a specific mismatching between these
two subsystems, e. g. even level of tension and widening.

5) In the clashing of maternal and infantile patterns.

A tendency towards an imbalance can be seen in infancy
when there is a deficiency in matching rather than mismatching, e. g. when high intensity is not structured by
shortening or widening is not backed by tension-flow adjustment.

Transitions

Some young infants find means of ameliorating clashes within themselves and between themselves and others. It is much more difficult to bring on balance where imbalance persists. Most infants need some help in learning to combine affine movement patterns to achieve equilibrium. In each record I have seen there were periodic alternations between clashing and harmony, balance and imbalance. As the ego takes over the control of motility one can see transitions from early to later forms of harmony or conflict, with or without the disappearance of the old when newer forms appear. What has been seen as clashes within subsystems is frequently transformed into clashes between them, with ensuing conflicts between the id and the ego.

It is understood that the ego gradually takes over the control of affects, but it is never in full charge of them as it is in charge of defense mechanisms or even more so of coping with reality. While we do not exclude the ego's influence upon the tension-and shape-flow attributes, we assume that the primary psychic regulation over these patterns is intimately connected with the regulation of physical needs, represented in the id. Thus, if there are clashes between these subsystems and the ego-controlled effort or shaping, we assume that there is a conflict between the id and the ego.

Clashes between subsystems which reflect <u>conflicts between the id and the ego</u> can be seen in:

1) The clashing between tension-flow and precursors of effort or effort. These can be a) general, as in the combination of high intensity and hesitation, or b) specifically dissonant, as in abrupt deceleration.

2) The clashing between shape-flow and shaping in directions or planes. These can be: a) general, as in unipolar bulging and moving across the body or b) specifically dissonant, as in unipolar caudal lengthening and ascending or bipolar hollowing and advancing.

Clashes between ego controlled movement patterns which suggest <u>conflicts in the ego</u>, are:

1) Vertical clashes [a) general, b) specific] between:

a) the heterogeneous elements of precursors of effort and effort, such as vehemence, combined with indirectness.

b) the homogeneous elements of precursors of effort and effort elements, as in the dissonant combination of vehemence and lightness.

Vertical clashes between:

a) the heterogeneous elements of shaping in directions and shaping in planes, such as pointing upward while retreating.

b) between the homogeneous elements of shaping in directions and shaping in planes, as in the dissonant combination of pointing upward while descending

2) Horizontal clashes [a) general and b) specific] between:

a) the heterogeneous elements of precursors of effort and shaping in directions, and the heterogeneous elements of effort and shaping in planes, exemplified by flexibility combined with retreating or by acceleration with enclosing.

b) the homogeneous elements of precursors of effort and shaping in direction, and the homogeneous elements of effort and shaping in planes, exemplified in the mismatched combination of channeling and moving sideways, or the mismatched combination of strength and spreading.

In vertical clashing we distinguish between a general incompatibility of aggression and indulgence, which fuse, separate and refuse in endless sequences and combinations, and a specific dissonance getween genetically related motor expressions of affect and of defenses or coping actions. In general clashing we may encounter movement expressive of aggressive feelings (like anger) and indulging benign defenses (like postponement) or vice versa of benign feelings combining with aggressive defenses or coping actions. We also encounter a clashing between defenses and coping actions as for instance in the combination of gentleness with acceleration. In specific clashes we encounter expressions of specific conflicts between dissonant affects and ego attitudes, as for instance using avoidance (flexibility) rather than isolation (channeling) to combat stubbornness (in which an even level of tension is needed to hold back) or between defenses and coping actions such as channeling and indirectness.

Parallel is the distinction between a general incompatibility of patterns serving withdrawal and those serving approach and a specific dissonance between genetically related motor expressions of self-feelings and of defenses against an object or relating to a constant object (Kestenberg et al, 1971). In general clashing, we may encounter movement expressive of grandiose expansive feelings combining with moving backward or retreating from what is ahead and a defensive protection against an enemy threatening from above, combined with making advances to the same person. In specific clashing, we encounter expressions of specific conflicts between dissonant self-feelings such as a feeling of constriction (narrowing) and defenses such as extending the boundaries of hospitality (moving sideways) or inviting a whole group of people to visit. There are also clashing expressions of specific defenses such as moving away from a source of danger with simultaneous advancing.

General vertical clashing implies a less organized type of antagonism among affects, defenses and coping mechanisms than the specific clashing which creates a dissonance between corresponding patterns. Clinically, we can distinguish between vague general conflicts and specific head-on collisions between exact opposites.

In horizontal clashing, we also distinguish between the clashing of heterogeneous elements and the mismatching of specifically related homogeneous patterns. Matching pertains to specifically paired related patterns of tension-flow and shape-flow (e.g., even flow and narrowing), of precursors of effort and shaping in directions (e.g., channeling and moving across), and of efforts and shaping in planes (e.g., directness and enclosing). General propositions are that tension-flow is structured by all three shape-flow systems--the bipolar, the unipolar and the shape-flow-design; that precursors of effort are structured by shaping in directions; and that effort is structured by shaping in planes. Over and beyond this general relationship between patterns and systems there is a more specific affinity between them, called matching, which underlies the correspondence of specific drives to specific drive objects, of specific defenses against drives to specific defenses against objects, and of specific coping mechanisms to specific shapes of relationships.

In transition to ego-controlled motility, specific affinities between tension and shape-flow are incorporated into the matching of effort and shaping elements. The function of selecting consonant and matching patterns is part of the ego's synthetic function. A dissonance or mismatching of related patterns is frequently the result of a failure of the synthetic function. An imbalance in which one of the related patterns is scanty or not in use prevents the operation of the synthetic function.

However, a flux from balance-to-imbalance-to-balance, from consonance-to-dissonance-to-consonance and from matching-to-mismatching-to-matching of patterns is comparable to the sequence of progression-regression-progression; all are signs of developmental progress.

Section IV

Gestures and Postures

(Appraising the ego- and the superego-organizations)

The focus of this section is not the transition from drive- to ego-dependent motility, but rather the evolution of movement controlled by the superego and the transition from ego- to superego-dominated patterns. The superego, a structure which differentiates from the ego in latency, has its precursors earlier in life. I shall try to trace precursors of the superego through the study of global postures and I will attempt to correlate integrated postural effort and shaping elements with superego functions. I shall use phrases of movement from the profiles of the three subjects as well as diagrams, constructed from the quantification of notated effort and shaping elements in gestures and postures, to demonstrate how one can deduce the influence of the ego and the superego on movement. Gesture-posture merging (Lamb, 1969) and clashing will be discussed as indicators of harmony and conflict between the ego and the superego. Matching and mismatching, in gestures and postures, will be discussed as indicators of harmony and conflict within the ego and superego respectively. Conflicts and imbalance will be differentiated.

a. The Merging and Clashing in Postures and Gestures

In the newborn we can see mass movement in which all the parts of the body are involved simultaneously or successively. These movements are rarely performed with the same pattern. In pathological cases and in normal infants under stress we can see the whole body stiffen or become limp. There are moments in which we can detect a shrinking or growing of the whole body, but these are few and far between. Perhaps the most striking total body involvement in certain patterns is seen in startles, in which free flow alternates with bound flow, and growing alternates with shrinking. When startles are inconspicuous or less pronounced, these patterns are only seen in the periphery or only in the upper extremities.

Transitions

Attuning and adjusting to his mother, who embraces
the infant's whole body during nursing, the baby learns
to centralize rhythms of tension- and shape-flow, and
thus involve his whole body in the service of a function.
In order to perform an isolated movement, such as turning
to the nipple, the infant learns to apply partial stabilization. Under conditions of partial stabilization during nursing or sucking from the bottle, the immobilization of the body gives support to the one part which must
be kept in motion, namely the sucking apparatus. Centralization of rhythms in the service of a function is
the prototype of postural movements; partial stabilization in the service of an isolated function is the prototype of movements in gestures. When we speak of postures
we primarily refer to patterns of effort or shaping in
which the whole body is engaged in supporting and carrying out a given motion element. When we speak of gestures, we refer to movement which can be seen in body
parts, such as arms, legs, trunk or head. Other parts of
the body can remain immobile or carry out other types of
gestures. For instance, the right arm may advance and
the left retreat, or both legs may kick while the fingers
fiddle.

Forerunners of mature postural changes in effort and
shaping are global postures in which either all parts of
the body are equally involved or the whole body acts as
one unit. They are primarily used for changes from one
position to another, as in turning, rolling, stooping,
rising, jumping or leaping.

When a young child uses his whole body to enclose an object, all of him seems to become one
with the object. His wish (coinciding with his
ideal) to totally possess is reflected in the global
posture of enclosing and perhaps in straining as
well. Reminded by the mother that he must share or
return the object, he may get a tantrum jumping up
and down with his whole body; he may try to hide
the object by stooping and decelerating as he begins to wind himself around the coveted possession.
When he gives in and returns the toy, he may suddenly spread out his arms and legs in a new global
posture that seems to indicate: "I have nothing,
you can have it."

Mature, integrated postural efforts and shaping in
planes are patterns which serve organized activity rather
than mere changes in position. In integrated postures,
all body parts, moving in continuity, support and enhance
one or more elements of motion. For example, in postural
advancing, one leg supports the body while the other proceeds forward and up in the sagittal plane. One arm may

90

come forward and up, covering either less or more space than the leg. In changing from one leg to another, the head, chest and one arm may already be ahead while the pelvis has not yet followed through. A child who has begun to walk frequently uses one limb at a time in several gestures or moves in global postures by putting the weight of his body on one foot and then another. Not all parts of the body are equally involved, as in adult postural strength, but they all contribute to the successful execution of a strong action. A child may develop strength by pulling himself up; if the strength is distributed equally in all parts of the body, which acts as a unit, this is not an integrated but a global posture. According to Lamb, an advanced integrated postural movement in shaping or effort does not become a dependable item in the child's movement repertoire until mid-latency. Yet, even at this time, there is little coordination between postures and gestures.

Partial stabilization of tension-flow isolates one part of the body from the rest[13] as a precondition for differentiated functioning via gestures. A flow regulation, based on proper functioning of tension- and shape-flow changes in the service of varying tasks, enables us to use the same part of the body for movement phrases composed of several gestures. An example of such a phrase is a sequence of reaching, grasping, bringing the object to the mouth and lowering it again. A regulation of tension- and shape-flow which distributes qualities of motion in various parts of the body enables us to perform coordinated actions through the use of simultaneous and successive gestures in different parts of the body. These regulations come into the service of the ego which uses them to govern the distribution of shaping and effort in single and multiple gestures in accordance with the reality principle. Gesticulation for the expression of feelings primarily uses tension- and shape-flow. When it serves communication, it employs shaping and/or efforts.

All effective work movements are composed of effort and shaping in planes. An example of multiple work-gestures, some isolated from each other but all acting in coordination, is right-handed writing with acceleration while spreading to the right, the left hand holding the paper in place with some strength, and the left arm enclosing the spatial area of the writing sheet. This type

---

13) In minimal brain damage, this isolation frequently fails. Associated movements (in German, "Mitbewegungen") of the left arm or leg occur when the child has been asked to move the right only.

of cooperative venture reflects the ego's differentiating
and coordinating functions and is dependent on the ego's
reality testing for the proper execution of a task.

The latency child practices the coordination, matching and harmonizing of efforts and shaping in gestures.
At first he uses more global postures than integrated
ones, and he tends to isolate gestures from postures. A
global postural movement appears to represent a merging
of id, ego and superego into one, not too well differentiated, unit. Integrated postural movement is seen in
early latency, especially in activities learned from
adults, but it is not too frequent. From mid-latency on,
when the superego has become more clearly differentiated,
the child becomes increasingly more capable of performing
in integrated postural patterns, but he still tends to
isolate postures from gestures.

In early latency Glenda would become totally immersed in bound flow when she forced herself to
remain at the table to finish her homework. Upon
completion of her last writing gesture, she would
pause very briefly and then suddenly leap away from
the table, her whole body committed to global advancing and acceleration in free flow. She seemed
to have given herself whole-hearted, unqualified
permission to hurry off to play.

Later in latency, she would show her impatience
in a sudden leg gesture when she wanted to leave
the table to play. This would be followed by bound
flow and channeling which restrained the offending
limb. An integrated postural hesitation, distributing itself in a graceful way through the body,
would ensue. The bound flow and channeling constituted an inhibition and an isolation of the gesture
from the postural movement. When she was leaving
the table, she rarely leapt in a global postural
acceleration, but rather would use an integrated
postural acceleration. She could use all parts of
her body judiciously in the service of hurrying (in
an ego syntonic way and in accordance with the
requirement of her superego--a superego which became
integrated into a meaningful whole). Her timing
became objective and her total body geared to con-
tend with time. Yet, her phrasing did not encompass
smooth transitions from an accelerating gesture to
an accelerating postural movement. Either a pause
or another pattern would interpose itself to isolate
gestures from postures.

In transition between latency and adolescence, iso
lation between gesture-and posture-patterns decreases.

Phrases of "gesture-posture-gesture" patterns begin to appear.

An eleven year old child hesitating on his way home may drag his feet in a series of leg gestures. Attracted by something he sees, he will advance and descend either in gestures or in a smooth gesture-posture phrase. He may then stop and remind himself that he must rush home and begin running with a postural acceleration which goes over into acceleration in a gesture. He may repeat this phrase with each gesture becoming a transition for the next postural acceleration. At one point, he may end the phrase with a decelerating gesture and begin to play with the object he found by throwing it up with some vehemence, but he cannot really be at peace with this game because it interferes with his obligation to get home on time. To make up for the delay he may make one sudden global leap forward and get back to sequences of gesture-posture-merging in acceleration and advancing. This time his transitions are composed of gestural retreat and a decrease in acceleration.

Analyzing the sequence described above, we discover at first a sequential organization in foot-dragging gestures and assume that it is ego-syntonic; the repeated use of hesitation appears to be an affirmation of a delaying defense. Picking up the object may be merely directed by the ego to satisfy the child's curiosity or it may also be reinforced by the ego-ideal, urging him to make sure that the object be inspected. Rather than continuing with a gesture of ascending, he stops, isolating the episode from his next postural acceleration. He begins to run from the bent-down position. It seems that the superego has intervened and has ordered the ego to do what is necessary to get home quickly. There is harmony between the ego and the superego, but with each gestural acceleration, there is a new reinforcement by the superego. This is expressed in the renewal of the postural acceleration. At one point, however, the ego takes over, as he institutes a decelerating gesture to finish off the previous phrasing. Disobediently, he plays with the object he found, and once more we see the preponderance of defensive patterns. Without transition, and once again isolating the ego from the superego, he leaps up with a global surrender and a wish for total atonement for the delay. The ensuing phrases are more complicated than any of the others. The retreat-gesture clashes with the advancing in gesture and posture, but it is used for recuperation and as a way of giving new impetus to acceleration and advancing. The ego's rebellious attitude is converted into a useful transition for actions, urged on by the superego, thus creating a compromise between the two psychic agencies.

As adolescence proceeds, gesture-posture-gesture phrases become more and more frequent, some merging patterns and some using either generally or specifically clashing movement qualities. Merging is a term, used by Lamb (1961, 1969) to indicate that the gesture and the following posture or vice versa were performed in the same pattern. There can be merging in one pattern and clashing in another. For instance, a direct gesture can extend into a direct postural motion, while at the same time, the lightness of the gesture is followed by strength in the postural motion. Non-merging or clashing can be seen when different or opposing patterns are used. For instance, advancing with hand and arm to greet someone and following through with the whole body not advancing, but ascending is a non-merging of a gesture into posture in advancing. Should the greeter who extended his arm follow through with a postural retreat without having isolated the gesture from the posture, a clashing between gesture and posture would occur. At the end of the retreating posture, the arm may advance again, which would constitute a clashing between posture and gesture. Sequences of merging, and clashing gesture-posture-gesture phrases reflect an organization in which a trial action in a gesture is followed by an approved action in a posture and ends in a gesture which limits the extent of commitment and approval (Kestenberg and Robbins, 1975). These phrases reveal various ways of problem solving through motor channels.

While the latency child has a stake in separating the ego from the superego, the separation between these structures weakens in early adolescence. Regression and progression, in their mutual relationship, are a characteristic of adolescent development. Uninterrupted, fluid sequences of merging and unmerging or clashing gestures and postures reflect the merging and unmerging and separation of the ego and the superego's functions, as they are practiced by the mover. The boundaries between the structures shift and become reestablished in variable ways, with a greater differentiation of some functions such as observing in the ego and the observing in the superego and a lesser differentiation of others, such as the idealization of the self and objects in the two structures. Conflicts become numerous, but there are also numerous and varying attempts to solve problems which lead into longer or shorter periods of harmony.

Adolescence exaggerates all conflicts. There are conflicts between the id and the ego. In movement we see them in the clashing of tension-flow and efforts and

94

of shape-flow and shaping, especially through dissonance.
In addition, there are pronounced subsystem clashes of
various shades of affect, defenses, coping actions and
manners of relating. Mismatching between tension and
shape-flow and between effort and shaping, creates the
many awkward moments that occur in the life of adolescents. Their feelings of anxiety or freedom to act are
often out of keeping with the image they have of themselves; their achievements are out of pace with their
self-esteem and their aspirations. The resulting con-
fusion calls for a reorganization, and it is the sequencing of merging, unmerging, clashing and merging
gesture-posture-gesture sequences that creates order out
of chaos, in movement.

In middle adolescence, postural movements increase
in frequency and tend to follow one another without
intervening gestures. Rapidly changing sequences of
dissonant and consonant, mismatching and matching postural
tension-flow-efforts and shape-flow-shaping attributes
and elements reflect the middle adolescent's rapid changes
in commitments. Conflicts and their resolutions arise
without preparations in trial actions (by initiating
gestures) and without testing the limits of the commitment
(by concluding gestures).

In late adolescence, gestures and postures become
well defined and phrases become more clearly differentiated into preparations, main themes and resolutions or
transitions into new actions. Postural patterns can be
part of preparations, resolutions or transitions, provided these adjuncts of the main theme also reflect
special commitments on the part of the mover.

In transition to adulthood, preferences for certain
types of phrasing become consolidated. What was once a
tendency to phrase in a series of gestures, with preferred beginnings and endings and endings in tension-
flow and shape-flow phrases, may be reproduced later in
typical phrases of specific gesture-patterns merging or
clashing with postural patterns in effort and shaping.

As an infant, Charlie tended to gradually increase and decrease his tension. In two phrases,
taken from the notation of his profile (see page
115) at the age of almost twenty, we see a tendency
to begin a phrase with deceleration and either keep
it up through the entire phrase or renew it in the
end-phrase. The tendency to increase tension and
then abate it also noted in one of the phrases
where the genetic successors of low and high tension,
lightness and strength follow the pattern of strength
appearing in the main theme and lightness at the beginning and the end. Charlie's high degree of cen-

95

tralization in infancy lives on in his present use
of many patterns in postural effort and his continuing need to have one postural effort follow another.

Perhaps it may be useful to analyze one of Charlie's
phrases in effort (See below and on p. 115) and another in
shape (see below and on p. 118) and examine the gesture-
posture-gesture sequences in the light of what we know
about his past.

In phrase B (below), Charlie's preparation consists of what might have been a gliding action in
bound flow, if not for the fact that he used gentleness rather than lightness and channeling instead of
directness. This highly loaded action merged into a
postural semi-gliding and was followed in the main
action by flow changes in bound flow with a renewal
of deceleration in a gesture merging into a posture
and culminating in another posture as a punch (see
glossary for a definition of gliding and punching and
other basic efforts), with a posture-posture clashing in time. In the resolution of the phrase, clashing occurred from posture to gesture in flow and in
time, strength disappeared and directness merged
from posture to gesture.

Sequences of harmony between the ego and superego are inferred from the gesture-posture merging.
These are followed by expressions of conflict within the superego (inferred from posture-posture
clashing in time), and end in an expression of conflict between the ego and superego regarding time
and flow, and a harmony regarding a direct approach
to space. Charlie could now assume a glide-like
gesture without feeling constrained and without
having to be defensive about it.

As an infant, Charlie's graduality clashed with
the abruptness of his mother, and he quickly learned
to adopt abruptness in response to her. Today's
conflict between the ego and the superego is a des-
cendent of this clash with his mother. In addition,
his mother has recently slowed down, and this too
may have had an influence on Charlie's time conflict.
This recent identification with his mother and the
continued identification with his slow father helped
Charlie to resolve his time conflicts some of the
time.

Since we know much less about Charlie's preferred
shape-flow attributes in infancy, we can say little
about the influence of congenital preferences for
certain shape-flow attributes upon his present phrasing in shaping. We note in phrase B, p. 118 (reproduced below), that he began with a downward movement and unipolar caudal shortening. In the main
theme, he bulged and advanced; then, moving postural-
ly, he lengthened symmetrically and then narrowed
asymmetrically while coming forward. There was some
merging, but no clashing, between gesture and posture.
In the resolution of the phrase he resumed his unipolar shortening and transformed the forward motion
into advancing in another posture. There was some
merging, but no clashing, between the main-theme and
the end-posture. In comparison with the effort phrase,
the shaping phrase showed much less richness. We
know from Charlie's profile that his shaping load-
factor was lower than that for effort and that he had
fewer clashes in gesture-posture shaping than in gesture
posture effort (p. 130). It is not surprising to
discover that Charlie's relationships were less complex than his dynamics, and his phrasing in shaping
(as seen in the representative sample) was correspondingly less varied than in effort.

Examining sequences of phrases in gestures and
postures, it is difficult to show a correlation between
each change in movement patterns and a specific change
in the psyche. The difficulty is similar to the one we
encounter when we try to extrapolate the influences of
the id, ego and superego from verbal phrases and sentences
used by a patient. Although I tried to avoid the pitfalls
of equating movement with thought or movement-patterns with
the psychic structures regulating them, I may have unin-
tentionally given the impression that I was translating
movement into language or into metapsychological concepts.
In addition, my experience in comparing the analysis of
movement phrases with the analysis of concomitant verbal-
ization is limited. The foregoing sample interpretations
of phrases must, therefore, be taken as suggestive of how
phrases in gesture-posture sequencing could be analyzed,
rather than standing as verified conclusions. It is
clear from my references to clinical impressions that I
used a general clinical assessment, rather than any direct
knowledge of what was going on in the mover's mind, to
test phrase interpretations. I find myself on safer

ground when I compare psychological assessments based on movement profiles (rather than on phrases) with assessments derived from conventional psychoanalytic investigative techniques. Comparisons have been made with Anna Freud's (1965) developmental profiles (Kestenberg, 1975), but more frequently with the less precise tools of the usual clinical assessment. In the following subsection, I shall attempt an appraisal of the relations between the ego and the superego through the interpretation of the gesture-posture ratio, revealed in the effort- and shaping-diagrams in the movement profile. The profiles of Glenda, Charlie and Nancy will provide us with illustrations showing how such an appraisal can be made. My assumptions have yet to be validated in a more formal way.

Gestures and Postures in Profiles (pp. 129-131)

The stronger the superego, the more power it has with which to subdue the ego. The weaker the superego, the less pressure it can exert on the ego. The superego's influence need not be invoked often; the ego can function for long stretches of time without pressure from the superego. This can happen when the ego rebels against superego demands and overrides its admonitions, or when it functions in a conflict-free manner without a need for the superego to intervene on its own behalf. We must also note that areas of influence of the superego are not evenly distributed. Each individual's conscience differs, pressing for conformance in some and giving in to the ego in other sectors of the internal code. Individual differences, expressed through movement, can be studied in the effort and shaping diagrams contained in profiles; that is, provided we accept the assumption that movement in gestures is regulated by the id-ego while postural movements are also under the influence of the superego. It is implied that the ego in its use of effort and shaping has assumed control over motor expressions of the id --the id's influence being operative in all actions.

It must be noted that the extent of the areas bounded by interrupted and dotted lines, indicating gestures and postures respectively, depends not on the number of actions notated, but on their load factor (L-F). The number of actions, listed above the diagrams (see ill. 4, 5 & 6, and profiles in the appendix), simply shows how many posture- and gesture- actions had been notated during the observation; it does not indicate whether these actions were highly loaded. The more patterns used per action, the higher the load factor. In the profile-diagrams, the loading of all notated actions is taken into consideration and the L-F on top of the diagram is an averaged, composite number. By comparing the load factors for gestures and postures, we infer how effective the influence of gesture patterns is in comparison to posture patterns. The more frequently an element is evoked in an action, the larger the area allotted to that element on the diagram. (For instance, in Nancy's profile, the most frequently encountered shaping, occurring alone or in combination with others is the element of spreading).

From the number of postural actions, we deduce the frequency with which the superego has been invoked; from the number of actions in gestures, we deduce how often the ego has controlled the movement in relative independence from the superego. The larger the area bounded by dotted lines, the stronger, we assume, the influence of the superego is; the larger the area bounded by interrupted lines, the stronger is the influence of the independently functioning ego. The overlap of these two areas represents a conflict-free sphere in which neither ego nor the superego are opposing one another. 14)

> Under the influence of her superego, Glenda diminished her aggression and reduced her opportunities for exposure to people (ill. 4a, 4b). This is inferred from the constriction of "fighting" effort elements, and of "open-shaped" shaping elements in postures, respectively. The abundance of acceleration, strength and directness, and of advancing, ascending and spreading in gestures seemed to express the ego's rebellion against the superego. There was a noticeable harmony between gestures and postures in enclosing. Descending and retreating became prominent in postures, while retreating hardly ever occurred in gestures. Clinical impressions confirmed the interpretations that Glenda's punitive superego had become weaker to the extent that she could aggressively demand and seek her mother's help, making herself dependent on her during her pregnancy; but her ego-ideal, though scantily evoked, was occasionally good enough to impose upon the ego the use of protective measures by retreating and by an increase of descending. These "closed-shaped" patterns safeguarded the middle and the lower part of her body against exposure to contact.

---

14) Lamb (1969) bases his assessment of business executives on this area of overlap. He refers to it as the sphere of gesture-posture merging.

Illustration 4

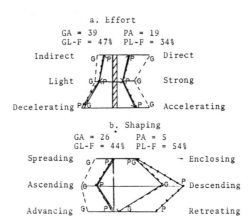

a. Effort
GA = 39   PA = 19
GL-F = 47% PL-F = 34%

Indirect ... Direct
Light ... Strong
Decelerating ... Accelerating

b. Shaping
GA = 26   PA = 5
GL-F = 44% PL-F = 54%

Spreading ... Enclosing
Ascending ... Descending
Advancing ... Retreating

Illustration 4. Diagrams representing the distribution of effort and shaping elements in Glenda's
latest profile. The areas of gestures are outlined
in interrupted lines; the areas of postures are outlined in dotted lines. Solid lines indicate the
area in which gestures and postures overlap.
GA = number of gesture-actions. PA = number of posture
                                     actions.
GL-F = load factor in gestures. PL-F = load factor in
                                        postures.

Giving up or diminishing a function when the superego is invoked, and retaining it when the ego frees itself from superego demands, are characteristic of neurotics
whose inhibitions are confined to certain important states,
such as pregnancy, or important events, such as an examination. However, even in those times, only a selected
function may be disturbed.

Under the influence of his superego, Charlie
tended to become inattentive and his capacity to
explore was reduced. This could be inferred from
the reduction of direct efforts and spreading elements of shaping in postures as compared to gestures (ill. 5a, 5b). A description of Charlie's
early learning difficulty and of his ability to
perform under optimal circumstances of reduced
pressure is included in the first volume of this

book. The conflict with his mother and teacher, discussed there, has become internalized. Charlie failed tests, but was attentive and interested when he was not constrained by guilt and shame. The conflict weakened Charlie's superego, but did not prevent it from expanding in other areas of functioning. Its strength as compared to the ego could be deduced from the effort load-factor of 56% in postures as compared to 48% in gestures. This did not pertain to that aspect of the superego which we call ego-ideal. The aspirations of the superego were reduced and weaker than Charlie's self-appraisal (see the low postural load factor of 38% and the higher gesture-load factor of 43% in shaping. The areas in which the superego was more influential than the ego could be deduced from the expansion of postural strength, acceleration and deceleration and advancing. Charlie's determination and his management of time have improved considerably under the guidance of his superego, and he has become very interested in advancing himself in the work he is doing at this time. Noticeable was the merging between gestures and postures in all closed-shaped patterns which suggests that he was at peace wth himself when he barred access to his body.

Illustration 5

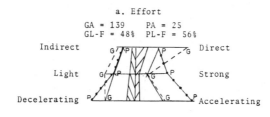

a. Effort

GA = 139   PA = 25
GL-F = 48% PL-F = 56%

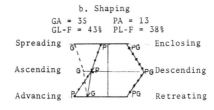

b. Shaping

GA = 35   PA = 13
GL-F = 43% PL-F = 38%

Illustration 5. Diagrams representing the distribution of effort and shaping elements in Charlie's latest profile.

Most of the records I have seen showed that efforts and shaping are used much less frequently in postures than they are in gestures. An occasional regression due to developmental changes or stress leads to a lowering of the frequency with which actions directed by the superego occur (see the small number of postural shaping-actions in Glenda's profile in ill. 4b) However, it is rather unusual to find a complete lack of postural patterns, or just a few among many gestures, in children over the age of eight. Such a finding in an adolescent or an adult suggests either a lack of progression or a regression in psychic differentiation.

During a two-hour observation of Nancy at the age of twenty (ill. 6), I notated 51 effort actions in gestures and only 7 in postures. No postural shaping was in evidence. However, the very high load factor in posture-effort (59%) indicated that its impact was of a very high order. Once Nancy came under the influence of a superego, she became highly influenced by it. The interview with Nancy confirmed the interpretation of the profile data. Nancy had internalized commands that she hurry and that she be determined. At the same time, she demanded of herself that she accommodate and yield to circumstances in her family, her social life and her work. Clinical data also confirmed the impression gained from the profile that Nancy's ego was constricted; without an internal pressure, all she could do with regularity was to combine whatever effort she used with acceleration. The absence of postural shaping suggested that Nancy had not internalized her ego ideal; for guidance, she looked to people around her (her immediate family) and to those above her (her older sister and her brother).

Illustration 6

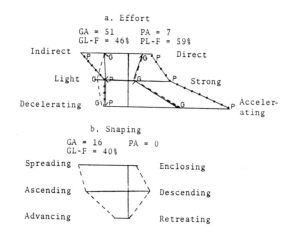

Illustration 6. Diagrams representing the distribution of effort and shaping in Nancy's latest profile.

In line with our investigation of the influence of earlier patterns on more advanced patterns, we must consider the question of what role the original predilections, identifications and developmental shifts played in the selection of postural patterns in the adulthood of our three subjects.

Charlie's original tendency to gradually become very intense presaged a preference for deceleration and strength. These are now more pronounced in postures than in gestures, but the same is true of acceleration, which had been enhanced by the motions of his mother and siblings. Nancy's original abruptness and high intensity has been transposed into acceleration and strength which are now much more noted in her few postural efforts than in her gestures. Glenda's newly developed directness is constricted in postural movement, but her acceleration, a descendant of her abruptness, is restricted as well. At the time of her pregnancy there was a decisive shift towards femininity with a concomitant

103

reduction of aggressive patterns. Further longitudinal studies are needed to determine the influence
of congenital traits, developmental shifts and
learning on postural effort and shaping. Such studies will also enable us to pursue further the correlation between postural patterns and superego
functions.

Matching and Mismatching, Balance and Imbalance Between

Effort and Shaping in Gestures and Postures

Our interpretations of effort and shaping in gestures
and postures were derived from comparisons of Movement
Profiles with Clinical Assessments. These can be summar-
ized as follows.

Efforts in gesture are motor expressions of ways in
which the ego deals with adaptation to reality. Shaping in
gestures are motor expressions of representations in the
ego of the self, functioning in relation to others. The
effort and shaping gesture-diagrams in the profile present
us with a survey of the distributions of these functions in
the ego. Inasmuch as there are six effort elements and six
shaping elements in the diagrams, they also contain a fair
representation of the distribution of more specific adaptive and object-oriented ego functions. By comparing the
gesture load-factor in effort and in shaping, we can
appraise which of the two ego functions, adaptive (a)
and object-oriented (o), has a greater impact on behavior.
The comparison of the amount of actions used is not
precise, but it can give us an idea as to the frequency
distribution of (a) and (o) in a sample.

Postural efforts are motor expressions of the involvement of all psychic agencies, including the punitive
superego, in adapting to reality. Shaping in postures,
used in the service of self-object relationships, indicates the involvement of all psychic agencies, including
the ego-ideal aspect of the superego. We are discussing
here only effort and shaping, which imply control over,
and incorporation of tension-flow and shape-flow respectively. It is assumed that the ego, in mediating between
the id and reality, has incorporated in its functions
derivatives of the id. It would take us too far afield
to compare the respective contributions of the id and the
ego (from comparisons of tension-flow with effort, and of
shape-flow with shaping). Neither is it possible here to
specify the intrasystemic conflicts that can be inferred
from the matching and mismatching of tension- and shape-
flow systems.

We define matching as the use of specifically re-

lated homogeneous patterns of effort and shaping, as for
instance strength with descending. When one pattern (e.g.
strength) is frequently used and the related pattern
(descending) is either absent or used infrequently, while
the clashing pattern (ascending) is readily available, we
assume that there is considerable mismatching (of strength
with ascending). However, if two related patterns are
well matched (e.g. acceleration with retreating, and one
of their polarities (advancing) is abundant and the other
(deceleration) scanty or absent, there is an imbalance
rather than a mismatching of specific patterns. In the
above example advancing is frequently performed without
deceleration. If shaping patterns are not balanced by
related effort patterns, we refer to it as "form without
content", or as expressive of relations to objects without the backing of dynamic qualities, revealed in effort.
If effort elements are not balanced by related shaping
elements (e.g. deceleration without advancing), the
structure for a dynamic action is missing; we assume that
a particular type of adaptation to reality developed without a relation to an object and is independent of objects.
While mismatching expresses a special type of conflict
either in the ego or in the superego, imbalance implies a
retardation or incompleteness of structure.

There is an explicit assumption that postural efforts are specifically concerned with adaptation and
that the superego, controlling them, addresses itself to
forbidden or permissible adaptive actions. Furthermore,
it is assumed that postural shaping is specifically concerned with relating to objects and that the ideal in
the superego, which controls postural shaping, addresses
itself to aspirations and denigrations of the self in
relation to objects.

The superego may be severe in its condemnation of
dealings with external reality, as evidenced in the
relation of postures and gestures in effort. At the
same time, it can be lenient as far as one's aspirations
and relations to objects are concerned, as seen in the
relation of postures and gestures in shaping. The reverse can also be true. Various aspects of the ego
ideal can by far exceed the demands made by the punitive
superego in regard to the ego's dealings with reality.

The following examples will illustrate how functions
of the superego can be studied through the appraisal of
matching and mismatching in postural effort and shaping.

Glenda used postural shaping rarely, while postural effort was relatively frequent (See Effort
P-actions [19] and Shaping P-actions [5] in Ill.4).
However, when postural shaping did make an appearance, it exerted a considerable influence upon her

actions, far in excess of that exerted by postural efforts (See Effort P L-F 34% and Shaping P L-F 54%). This suggests that her punitive superego was invoked more often, but her ideal superego, when operative, had a greater impact upon her.

Glenda's recent curtailment of postural "fighting" efforts was not matched by a corresponding reduction of postural shaping elements. Descending increased and retreating was introduced as a major postural component. In contrast, among the open-shaped postural elements, ascending decreased and spreading and advancing were not used at all, revealing the conflict between seeking and curtailing of self-exposure. My clinical impression was in accord with the interpretation that Glenda's ego-ideal has shifted focus from an optimistic, lofty, forward looking tendency in the ego to an attitude of protectiveness, especially related to the lower a..d middle parts of her body. However, the aspiration to become protective could not be sustained by a comparable amount of aggression, creating an imbalance in the superego, whereby protectiveness was held up as an ideal but, not backed by punitive measures. A noticeable mismatching of postural deceleration with retreating revealed a conflict between an injunction to slow down and an encouragement to retreat.

There was a greater general correspondence between effort and shaping in gestures, indicating a greater harmony in the ego than in the superego. However, ego-disharmony could also be noted a minor imbalance in the areas of directness-enclosing and major ones in descending-strength and in acceleration-retreating. The latter was an aftermath of Glenda's longstanding conflict which made her rush ahead in a counter-phobic way. It was not surprising that so many of Glenda's conflicts concerned timing, an area in which she had clashed with her mother.

Charlie's shaping in gestures was neither as frequent nor as complex as his efforts (35 shaping- and 139 effort-actions; shaping load-factor of 43% and effort load-factor of 48%). We interpret these data to mean that his self-appraisal was lower than his capabilities warranted. Judging by the low load-factor in postural shaping (38%), his aspirations seemed to be even simpler than his self-appraisal. In postural shaping, Charlie considerably reduced his old-time-favored spreading, and his newer propensity for ascending decreased.

The assumption that Charlie's superego not only curtailed his attentiveness but also lowered his capacity to explore and look up to and be guided by models (inferred from the postural restriction of directness and of spreading and of lightness and ascending) has been clinically verified. His learning problem is largely due to a conflict between the ego and the superego, but a conflict in the ego persists. The mismatching of directness with spreading is reflected clinically in the fact that he spreads his attention to details instead of confining it to specific issues. An imbalance in the ego stems from Charlie's wish to show determination (through descending) without sufficient strength to back it up. From the almost flawless matching of postural effort and shaping patterns, we infer that Charlie's learning inhibition is sanctioned by a harmonious interaction of his punitive and his ideal superego. An imbalance in the superego, deduced from frequent postural accelerations not balanced by enough retreating is borne out by the fact that Charlie's involvements in accelerating his progress are frequently confused. His ideal is to advance but he cannot structure acceleration with looking back in order to appraise from where the best type of progress could be made. Flashes of insight, derived from learning from the past, are few and far between.

Although determined and hurried in her efforts to achieve, and feeling guilty when she did not, Nancy has not yet developed an ego-ideal that could be incorporated into her superego (See the lack of postural shaping in Ill. 6). Nancy's conflicts between the ego and the superego (about aggression and indirectness) were strong, but infrequent. Except in three small areas (inferred from the matching of direct efforts and enclosing in shaping, from scanty strength and descending, and from deceleration and advancing--all in gestures) there was little harmony in the ego. Judging from the relatively large areas of spreading and advancing, and the incongruously small areas of "indulging" efforts, and by the large area in accelerating and a complete lack of retreating, we would think that there is more than an imbalance, perhaps a disorder in the ego, rather than a conflict. It almost seems that each of the ego functions (coping with reality and relating to objects) has developed independently. There is no structure for Nancy's inordinate need to rush, and there is insufficient ability to accommodate to reality to back the expansiveness of the ego (in seeking contact with what is around her and above her). Her identification with her sister and her mother, and her emulation of their quest for contact with supernatural powers, are met by too little sub- stance in her accommodation to the environment. Since her development has been considerably delayed and still proceeds, there is hope that she may still transform her yearnings for exposure to contact into an ideal that can be incorporated into the superego. The ensuing balance in the superego may have a beneficial effect on the restoration of balance in the ego. Perhaps if her need to be loved can be fulfilled, she may develop sufficiently intense loving attitudes to counteract her aggression and to introduce aspirations into her conscience.

In contrast to Glenda's propensity for intra- systemic conflict and imbalance in the superego, Charlie's superego has achieved a good balance despite the fact that the degree of his punitive- ness by far exceeds his aspirations. His learning problems are upheld by conflicts between the ego and the superego and by an additional conflict in the ego. Nancy's punishing superego is new, rarely invoked, but strong. However, there is no evidence in her profile that an ego-ideal has been incorp- orated in the superego. This and the considerable imbalance in her ego suggests a deviant rather than a neurotic development, such as we find in Glenda and Charlie.

Charlie's propensity for centralization may be at the core of the good integration of his superego. Nancy's excessive stabilization may have been the beginning of an arrest that prevented the develop- ment of the superego at the appropriate time. Glenda's relatively good attunement and identifica- tion with her mother had its repercussions during her pregnancy, with the superego increasing protective- ness and decreasing her native inclination to acceler- ate. Charlie's external conflicts with his mother and sibling were internalized and manifested them- selves in conflicts between the ego and the superego. Nancy's deviant, jarring tension-flow rhythms were and still are at the core of her developmental im- balance.

While gesture-posture-merging may be used for the study of transitions from ego to superego-domina- ted patterns, the matching and balance in gestures and postures respectively can become the source for an investigation of differential contributions to the ego and superego respectively, in early development.

Four Factors in the Transition from Drive- to Ego Dependent Motility

In comparing the movement profiles at the end of adolescence with those reported in its beginning, one can find many changes which have developed over the period of maturation into near adulthood. Nevertheless, the areas of consistency which can be seen in the transitions from drive-to ego-dependent motility are numerous. They can be distinguished from many other variables as the factors which can be used for the prediction of later traits from earlier predispositions. Four such factors are listed here, with the understanding that it is easier to reconstruct than to predict.

1) Early preferences for certain rhythms of tension-flow are preserved in later rhythm-constellations. As interpreters of movement we can say that one can foretell what drive components will tend to participate more than others in future combinations of drives and drive-derivative behavior. One could have said, for instance, that phallic drive components would give a special tinge to Glenda's personality and, that Charlie's inner-genital drives would qualify the aims of other drives and would have an integrative effect upon his psychic structure. In the future, one may be able to make predictions about the development of relations to objects from early constellations of shape-flow and shape-flow-design rhythms.

2) One can foretell preferences for certain forms of organization from early prevalences of certain organizing influences, interdependent with rhythms of tension-flow. In Glenda's case, one could have predicted biphasic functioning; in Charlie's case a superior capacity for integration; and in Nancy's case repetitiousness and imbalance.

3) One can predict that tension-flow attributes which are contained in originally preferred rhythms have a specific relationship to later maturing ego-controlled efforts and their precursors; similarly, one can expect a progressive relationship between preferred shape-flow attributes and the later maturing ego-controlled shaping in directions and in planes of space. This implies that temperament or persistent modes of affect-regulation can influence future choices of defenses and coping mechanisms, and that self-feelings can selectively promote certain forms of approach and relating to objects.

4) On the basis of various early affinities and clashes within and between tension-flow and shape-flow of the

infant and his mother, one may be able to foretell the degree and type of harmony versus conflict which facilitate or impede development. Intrasystemic conflicts in the ego may have their antecedents in clashes of tension- and shape-flow attributes. Perhaps one can attempt to predict future trends in the superego from the appraisal of its precursors, as they are expressed in centralized and global total body movements in infancy and childhood.

CHAPTER 7

METHODS OF NOTATION THAT PERMIT OBJECTIVE
DIFFERENTIATION BETWEEN RHYTHMIC DISCHARGE
OF TENSION AND THE MORE MATURE COMPONENTS
OF MOVEMENT WHICH SERVE COMPLEX EGO FUNC-
TIONS

There are two methods of free-hand notation: one
traces changes in tension-flow, and the other traces
changes in the design of shape-flow. A sample of tension-
flow notation is reproduced in Illustration 7. For samples of shape-flow design notation, see Illustration 10,
p. 116.

Tension-flow tracings are scored in two ways: a) in
accordance with the classification of rhythms and b) in
accordance with the classification of tension-flow attributes in symbols (see Illustrations 7a, b).

a) The <u>rhythmic units</u> and their <u>abbreviations</u> are:

o = "oral" (sucking)   os = "oral-sadistic" (biting)

a = "anal" (twisting)   as = "anal-sadistic"(straining)

u = "urethral" (running)   us = "urethral-sadistic" (run-
                                             stop-go)
f = "feminine" or "inner-   fs = "feminine"- or "inner-
    genital" (undulant)   genital-sadistic" (swaying)

p = "phallic" (jumping)   ps = "phallic-sadistic"(leaping)

The symbols for tension-flow attributes, are the
same as Laban's effort symbols. To distinguish them from
effort we encircle them.

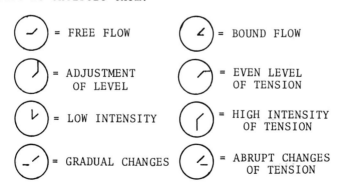

= FREE FLOW		= BOUND FLOW
= ADJUSTMENT OF LEVEL		= EVEN LEVEL OF TENSION
= LOW INTENSITY		= HIGH INTENSITY OF TENSION
= GRADUAL CHANGES		= ABRUPT CHANGES OF TENSION

Methods of Notation

Readers familiar with Laban's effort symbols should not find it difficult to learn to read our notation. For others, this provides a glimpse of the symbols we use.

Illustration 7

A sample notation of tension-flow from Glenda's record is scored as follows:

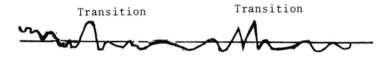

a) Scoring of rhythmic units:

> o,os,a,o,a,o,osf,a,os,osp,op,osp,us3,au,of,
> f2,fp2,ps4,os,asf,usf,o,a,af,osf

b) Scoring of tension flow attributes in symbols:

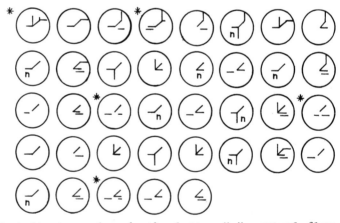

Asterisk indicates rebound, the letter "n" neutral flow.

Illustration 7. A sample notation and scoring from the most recent profile of Glenda. Note the phallic rhythms with their abrupt increases and decreases in tension which occur in transitions from one phrase to the next.

When the same rhythmic unit repeats itself in succession, the number of repetitions is indicated by a
numeral. Combinations of rhythmic units (mixed rhythms)
in the sample are: osf,osp,op,osp,au,of,fp2,asf,usf,af
and osf. There are 20 pure rhythms and 12 mixed. The
ratio of libidinal to sadistic type rhythms in pure
rhythms is 10:10 and in mixed rhythms is 16:6. The
ratio of component rhythms oral:anal:urethral:feminine:
phallic, in pure rhythms is 7:4:3:2:4 and in mixed
rhythms is 6:3:2:8:5.

Rhythmic units are quantified and projected onto a
diagram in such a way that one can distinguish pure from
mixed rhythms and easily see the proportions of various
rhythmic units noted during one observation session (see
Illustration 8).[15]

Illustration 8

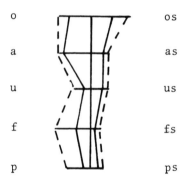

Illustration 8. Diagram of the rhythm distribution from
Glenda's latest profile. The vertical line divides the
"sadistic" from the "libidinal" type rhythms. The solid
lines indicate the frequency of pure rhythms and the interrupted lines indicate the frequency of mixed rhythms.
The only significance of the peripheral outlines on the
right and left sides is to present a gestalt of the diagram of pure (____) and mixed (---) rhythms.

---

15) For details of scoring, see Movement Profile Scoring,
    by J. Berlowe (1972), available through Child Develop-
    ment Research.

Methods of Notation

Tension-flow attributes are quantified and projected on diagrams (see Illustration 9) which were devised by Lamb (1965) for effort-shape representation.

Illustration 9

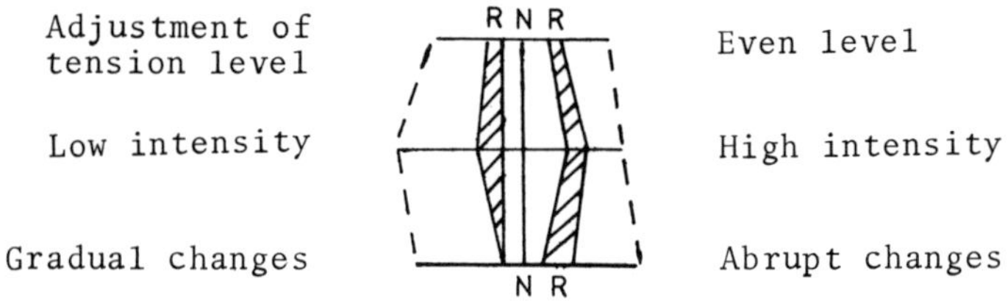

Adjustment of tension level		Even level
Low intensity		High intensity
Gradual changes		Abrupt changes

Free flow: Bound flow = 187:284

Illustration 9. <u>Diagram representing the distribution of tension-flow attributes from Glenda's latest profile.</u> The vertical line divides the "fighting" type on the right from the "indulging" type of attributes on the left. The peripheral lines, by their interrupted quality, indicate that the whole diagram pertains to movement in gestures. They also help to denote the Gestalt of the diagram. Changes in free and bound flow are counted separately and noted in their proportion. Shaded areas indicate the frequency with which attributes can be noted in neutral flow (N). The lined areas next to N indicate the frequency of rebound (R)--a slight reduction of a quality followed by an increase--which reveals the degree of resiliency.

Effort elements are written in symbols originated by Laban (1947):

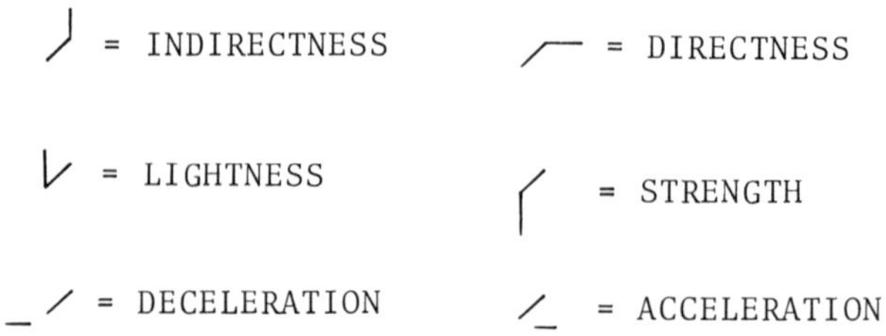

⌐ = INDIRECTNESS   ⌐ = DIRECTNESS

⌐ = LIGHTNESS   ⌐ = STRENGTH

⌐ = DECELERATION   ⌐ = ACCELERATION

Precursors of effort elements are written in the following symbols which were modified after Laban:

⌐ = FLEXIBILITY   ↗ = CHANNELING

↙ = GENTLENESS   ∫ = VEHEMENCE

↙ = HESITATION   ↗ = SUDDENNESS

FREE AND BOUND FLOW ARE ╱ AND ∠ RESPECTIVELY.

A sample notation of recent phrases by Glenda follows:

A) (╱⇢) ∠ ⤵⇢ (↓⇢)

B) (⸚⌐) ╱ ⤝ ╱ ∠ ⤸ (∠)

Preparations and endings of phrases are bracketed.

It remains to be added that notation also considers which patterns have been observed in gestures only (as above) and which appeared in postures or have merged from gestures into postures. Postural patterns are enclosed in squares. When a gesture merges into a posture it is indicated by an arrow. Two sample notations from Charlie's latest profile illustrate gesture-posture notation.

A) (↓)↗ᴾ ⊡ (↓)

B) (↙)↗ᴾ ∠ ∠↗ᴾ ⊡ (⤸)

Methods of Notation

Shape-flow-design is written in successive notation of pathways from the near- to the reach-zone and vice versa (see p. 40). It is scored in symbols, identical with shaping symbols and encircled to distinguish them from the latter.

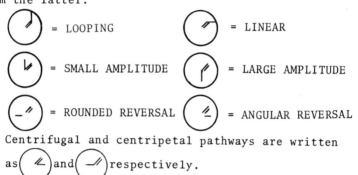

Centrifugal and centripetal pathways are written as and respectively.

Illustration 10

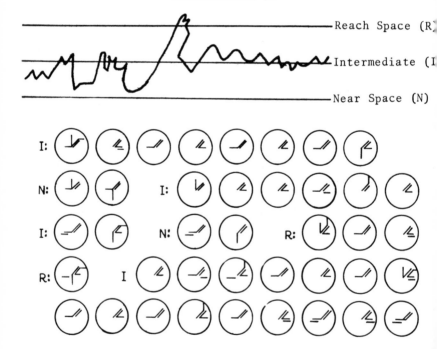

Illustration 10. A sample notation and scoring from the most recent profile of Nancy

116

Bipolar and unipolar shape-flow and shaping in directions and in planes are written in symbols, quantified and also projected in diagrams.

Bipolar Shape-Flow Attributes are written in symbols modified from Laban and Lamb (see also Cecily Dell, 1970):

∿⫽ = WIDENING   ⦘⌐ = NARROWING

⊢⫽ = LENGTHENING   ⫽⌐ = SHORTENING

⟋⫽ = BULGING   ⦘⟋ = HOLLOWING

Unipolar Shape-Flow Attributes are written in the following symbols which are also modified from Laban and Lamb:

⟵⫽ = LATERAL WIDENING   ⦘⟋ = MEDIAL NARROWING

⌞⫽ = CEPHALAD LENGTHENING   ⫽⌐ = CAUDAL SHORTENING

⦘⌞ = CEPHALAD SHORTENING   ⌐⫽ = CAUDAL LENGTHENING

⟋⫽ = ANTERIOR BULGING   ⦘⟋ = POSTERIOR HOLLOWING

⫽⟋ = ANTERIOR HOLLOWING   ⌐⫽ = POSTERIOR BULGING

Shaping in Directions is written in symbols, modified from Lamb and Laban:

⟋ = SIDEWAYS   ⟋⟶ = ACROSS THE BODY

⇑⫽ = UPWARDS   ∫⫽ = DOWNWARDS

⟋⫽ = FORWARDS   ⫽⟶ = BACKWARDS

GROWING AND SHRINKING ARE ⟋ AND ⟍ RESPECTIVELY.

Shaping in planes is written in symbols originated by Lamb:

⟋ = SPREADING   ⟋⟋ = ENCLOSING

⎣⫽ = ASCENDING   ⎡⫽ = DESCENDING

⫽⫽ = ADVANCING   ⫽⫽ = RETREATING

A sample notation of shape-flow-shaping phrases, from recent observations of Charlie, follows:

Before closing this section, it is important to stress that, to some degree, all movement patterns are operative at once in the adult. However, some movement patterns become distinct enough for notation while others are not recognizable and are therefore not notated. In addition, it is impossible to notate by freehand tracing and by the use of symbols at the same time. For some notators, it is impossible to notate efforts and shaping at the same time. Lamb recommends that they be done separately. Although film distorts movement, with careful technique it is possible to notate from film and thus obtain samples of all patterns from one and the same sequence. Research on notations from films is still in progress.

CHAPTER 8

PREDICTION AND OUTCOME

This study has been undertaken with the expressed
purpose of finding ways and means to notate and classify
movement patterns and correlate them with general behavioral data. This aim has been largely fulfilled. As
is frequently the case, our new discoveries and techniques necessitate further research projects. The correlations of movement profiles with psychological profiles should be validated on a larger scale (Kestenberg,
1975). There is a need for new longitudinal studies
which will rely on movement profiles of mother and child,
begun at birth or, even better, prenatally. The notation
of fetal movements promises to be a fruitful method for
the appraisal of the fetus and the mother. It is too
early to say what kind of predictions will be valid in
prenatal research. In a previous chapter, I have listed
several factors which may facilitate predictions in the
neonatal phase or in the early months of infancy. However, as is true of predictions made in psychoanalysis,
it is much easier to state at the end of a study what
predictions should have been made at its beginning than
to predict correctly in the beginning. I have learned
what predictions should not be made from observations of
movement patterns. It is not possible to anticipate the
occurrence of specific syndromes, such as strong penis
envy or a giving up of mother attachment in favor of the
father (p. 21 first volume, 1965). The greatest obstacle
to predictions is the lack of foresight regarding future
environmental conditions, such as the birth of Glenda's
brother when she was four years old.

General predictions were useful and were more often
substantiated than not, as for instance: "The congenitally
preferred rhythms...would be discernible in whole or in
part, with or without modification ... The preferred
motor rhythms of early infancy would be modified by maturation as well as by interaction with maternal...patterns...
Preferred rhythms...enhanced by the environment would...
become discernible in...temperament...(and)...would...
influence character..." (pp. 20-21 first volume, 1965).
The next statement, which predicted specific conflicts and
corresponding pathology from clashes between maternal and
infantile rhythms, was too broad and did not consider the
many variables which together conspire to form a specific
syndrome.

Prediction and Outcome

        Implicit in further attempts at prediction was the
idea that preferences for certain rhythms constitute a
readiness for a fixation in a specific drive organization.
One of the principal outcomes of this study is the discovery that there are pure, well differentiated and mixed
rhythms. Original preferences are frequently preserved
in mixed rhythms, and from the distribution of mixed
rhythms we can judge whether there is a fixation in a
given drive constellation. For instance, in Charlie's
profile (p.130) inner-genital rhythms are more frequent
in mixed rhythms than in pure and oral rhythms decreased
in proportion. This suggested an inner-genital type of
fixation.

        Preferred attributes of tension-flow and of shape-
flow may persist in their original form and/or may influence the selection of the more advanced movement elements. Persistence of preferred tension-flow attributes
and the traces they leave in precursors of effort and
effort proper are all indications of a type of fixation
which accounts for the individuality of temperament and
character traits. Further studies of the developmental
line from shape-flow attributes to shaping of space are
needed to appraise the nature of fixations and regressions
in regard to modes and styles of early and later relating.

        Many patterns have been notated, scored and inter-
preted since the onset of this study. Although we have
learned how some defense mechanisms are aided or represented by precursors of effort and directional shaping
(Kestenberg, 1979), we suspect that others may be represented in efforts and in shaping in planes. For instance,
retreat is a pattern of shaping in the sagittal plane;
moving backwards is a directional pattern. Both are
frequently used as responses to external danger. Through
a detailed description and scrutiny of certain combinations
of patterns, we sometimes discover forms of defenses which
have not been familiar to us. On the other hand, we have
not definitively identified patterns or combinations of
movement patterns which are operative in such specific
defenses as denial. We have scrutinized changes in the
shape of the body and have correlated them to early and
more advanced forms of relating to stimuli and objects.
However, we know much less about the way relationships are
expressed through movements than we know about the motor
expression of drives, defenses and adaptations.

        Our difficulty may in part be due to the fact that the
classification of relationships has not been as clearly
differentiated as the classification of drives and defenses (for a notable exception, see Gottschalk, 1968).
Nevertheless, the attempt to interpret various patterns
of shape-flow **has** led to a new conceptualization about

the role of motion factors in narcissism and masochism
(Kestenberg and Marcus, 1977), and about the development
of early ideation regarding the "self" and "others"
(Kestenberg, 1974). The appraisal of differences between effort and shaping in gestures and postures helped
us to make some inroads in the understanding of the influence of the superego and the ego-ideal on the selection of postural patterns.

An important discovery which clarified certain features of the motor behavior of Nancy and Charlie in their
infancies, was the observation and notation of neutral
flow of tension. Its occurrence signifies the use of deanimation as a method of dealing with drives. It is interesting that a certain degree of deanimation is used by
everybody, not only in states of tiredness or illness,
but also during adaptive activities which are then performed automatically with a mechanization of affect.
Neutral shape, which can be seen in the shapelessness of
autistic children, was either not in evidence in this
study, or was not recognized.

Among the many insights gained from this longitudinal study, the following findings should be emphasized:

The discovery of early types of organization suggested the possibility that certain rhythms of tension-
flow carry with them a propensity for certain types of
organization whose core remains the same from infancy to
adulthood. I refer here to Glenda's biphasic functioning;
to Charlie's capacity for centralization, which formed the
basis for the highly developed integrative function of his
ego, and presaged the balance in his superego; and to
Nancy's dysrhythmia which may have been the antecedent of
the imbalance in her ego.

The study of Glenda's movements during her courtship
and her pregnancy showed with great clarity that both,
but especially the latter, are adult developmental phases
with their specific characteristic forms of progression
and regression (Kestenberg, 1976).

Charlie's intersystemic conflicts, traceable from
early clashes with his mother, illustrated the influence
of congenital preferences, and maternal ·responses to them,
on the development of the superego.

A valuable insight was gained from the fact that,
in adolescence, Nancy caught up on some of the patterns
which she had missed in early development. Despite her
vulnerable disposition and the early deprivation from
which she suffered, maturation and new, improved environmental conditions made it possible for her to enter into

121

new, progressively more differentiated phases of development.

We have learned a great deal about combinations of patterns which harmonize or clash and create balance or imbalance. The clashing and the mismatching of qualities belonging to the two systems of movement, the clashing and the dissonances within a system, and the clashing of gestures and postures in effort and shaping presented us with the opportunity to explore in great detail intra-systemic and intersystemic conflicts, as they reveal themselves in movement. In addition, we were able to distinguish between conflict and imbalance.

Because our methods allowed us to study very early manifestations of harmony and clashing in the infant, himself and in relation to his mother, they opened up the possibility of gaining insight into some aspects of the id and the body-ego which are difficult to understand through purely verbal conceptualizations. However, the complexity and multitude of patterns and their combinations, which can be noted in movement, make us well aware of the fact that the study of harmony and conflict alone will take years of concentrated research.

MOVEMENT PROFILE (MP)

Notation, Scoring and Construction of Diagrams

Tension-flow is notated by a continuous tracing of tension-changes on paper. Shape-flow-design is notated by a continuous tracing on paper of the pathways traversed in space. All other patterns are notated in symbols adapted from Laban's (1947) effort notation.

Tension-flow is scored in two ways:

1) We assign to each successive form in the curve the appropriate name of a rhythmic unit, such as "o" for "oral" or "p" for "phallic". Computation of the number of rhythms scored in the pure and in the mixed variety is followed by a distribution of the rhythms - in accordance with their frequency in the record - and its transposition in percentages of the total on a diagram. Solid lines delimit pure rhythms and broken lines the mixed rhythms. Mixed rhythms are also listed separately to allow the profile-interpreter to survey the mixtures without having to look at the raw material.

2) We assign symbols to each tension-flow-attribute and to each element of free and bound flow, computing the frequency of their respective occurrences and projecting the ratio of attributes in such a way that the load-factor is represented (the method used was devised by Lamb [1961]). The ratio of free and bound flow is listed separately.

Shape flow-design is scored by assigning symbols to each change in the pathway of movement and to each centrifugal and centripetal movement and proceeding as above to construct the diagram. However, for this pattern the data are further subdivided into three sections: "N" for near space, "I" for intermediate space and "R" for reach-space. The subdivision is represented in the diagram.

All patterns, notated in symbols, (Precursors of effort, effort, bipolar and unipolar shape-flow, shaping in directions and in planes), are computed and distributed on the basis of their load-factor on diagrams comparable to the diagram of tension-flow attributes, described above.

All except the rhythm diagram, which has five lines, have three horizontal lines, divided by a vertical line. On the left side of the page are reproduced all diagrams representing patterns used for coping with the internal and external forces (tension-flow, precursors of effort and effort). On the right side of the page are reproduced all diagrams representing relatedness to environmental objects (such as air or temperature), to stimuli of a discrete nature, to respective positions of the person and the object, and to the multidimensional quality of self- and objects. The left side of the page can be referred to as the "effort-side" and the right as the "shape-side".

Each diagram has a right and a left side, divided by a vertical line. On the "effort-side", the right side of the diagram represents elements and attributes which are encompassed under the general heading of Laban's "fighting" qualities; on the "shape side", the right side of the diagram represents elements and attributes which can be subsumed under the heading "closed-shape". On the "effort-side", the left side of the diagram represents elements and attributes which are encompassed under the general heading of Laban's "indulging" qualities; on the "shape-side", the left side of the diagram represents elements and attributes which can be subsumed under the heading "open-shape". Free and bound flow, growing and shrinking, centrifugal and centripetal pathways are not included in the diagram, but listed separately.

The upper line in each three-line-diagram refers, on the effort-side, to patterns of approach to space or affine attributes, and on the shape side, to changes in the horizontal plane and affine designs. The middle line of the diagram refers, on the effort-side, to patterns dealing with gravity or affine attributes, and on the shape-side, to changes in the vertical plane and affine designs. The lowest line of the diagram refers, on the effort-side, to changes in time, and on the shape side, to changes in the sagittal plane and affine designs.

In the rhythm diagram, rhythms are listed from above to below in a sequential order representing the sequence of the developmental phases in which they are most prominent. The polarities in the rhythm diagram are "libidinal", represented on the left, and "sadistic", represented on the right.

To the side of the rhythm-diagram, we write the ratio of the rhythms computed in pure and mixed varieties, and the ratio of "libidinal" to "sadistic" rhythms found in each. Above each of the three-line-diagrams we note the ratio of free to bound flow, growing to shrinking or centrifugal: centripetal movement, as well as the gain expense ratio. The latter compares the number of attributes or elements used with the number of flow changes.

Above each three-line-diagram, we also list the number of actions found in the record. Each action must contain one or more attributes or qualities of a pattern. Bound flow, centrifugal movement or growing of shape are examples of motion qualities which are not called actions. Strength, enclosing or widening are all actions, computed for the diagrams of effort, shaping in planes or shape-flow, respectively.

Interpretation of the Profile

Although the MP has been geared for an optimal correlation with Anna Freud's developmental assessment (1965), it can be interpreted in general terms, based on the understanding of the patterns of movements whose distribution is represented in the MP.

A general description of the body attitude precedes all diagrams. In it can be listed all items which characterize the habits and movement of a person, which become apparent without notation. From the way the body is aligned, we can deduce how a particular developmental phase has contributed to the formation of the individual's body-image (Kestenberg, 1975).

From the rhythm-diagram, we can deduce how various needs, common to the human species, are distributed and we can reconstruct which developmental phase has been of greater importance in exaggerating some of the needs and reducing others.

From the tension-flow-attribute diagram, we gain a survey of the distribution of basic affective reactions which belong to the sphere of responses to safety and danger.

From the bipolar shape-flow diagram, we gain insight about a person's ability to express qualities of comfort and discomfort, and from the unipolar shape-flow-diagram we deduce how a person tends to react to discrete stimuli which either attract or repel him.

From the shape-flow-design diagram we can deduce in which part of the personal space the mover likes to move best, and we can further see which of the patterns, representing civility versus rudeness, are employed more frequently than others in the respective spatial zones.

From the precursors of effort-diagram, we can gain some insight as to how an individual reacts to danger.

This also applies to the learning situation, in which the unknown--the yet to be learned--belongs to the sphere of danger, in a broad sense of the word.

From the diagram of directional shaping, we conclude which directions had been preferred during the time of observation. It gives us a measure of understanding as to how the subject localizes objects and approaches the spatial expanse around him by creating lines of demarcation. These lines are also used for self-protection and are important landmarks in the structuring of the unknown experienced in learning.

From the diagram of efforts, we appraise the styles of and the ratio between the individual's attention, intention and decision-making processes. From the diagram on shaping in planes we appraise the styles of and the ratio between the individual's range of exploration, confrontation and anticipation functions (see first volume, 1967).

By comparing the diagrams on the left with those on the right, we gain insight into the degree of harmony or clashing between dynamic patterns and their structure. By comparing diagrams on the same side of the page, we gain insight as to the degree of harmony and conflict between patterns relating to the inside and the outside of the body.

By comparing the distribution of patterns in gestures with those in postures, we gain insight into the differences between functioning with a low or a high degree of motivation, or into the limits of functioning under conditions of partial versus total commitment.

To take into account phrasing and sequencing of patterns, we must appraise the raw data. If possible, we must look at the raw material also to see whether we can find instances of affinities and clashing during simultaneous notation of different patterns. This can be done for effort, shaping and attributes of all patterns notated in symbols.

1.

VERTICAL AFFINITIES AND CLASHING
WITHIN THE TWO MOVEMENT SYSTEMS

I. Movement System: Effort   II. Movement System: Shape [16)
   Composed of the Subsystems: Composed of the Subsystems:
   Tension-Flow Attributes;   Shape-Flow (Bipolar, Uni-
                                  polar and Design) Attributes;
   Precursors of Effort;   Shaping in Directions;
   Effort Elements.   Shaping in Planes Elements.

   a) General Affinity or Clashing Using Heterogeneous
      Attributes 17) and Elements

      Between "fighting" or   Between "closed-shaped" or
      between "indulging"   between "open-shaped" at-
      attributes and ele-   tributes and elements.
      ments.

      i. Within Individual Subsystems

          Examples: Examples:
            Affine low inten-   Affine bipolar widen-
            sity and graduality   ing with bipolar bulg-
                                   ing.
            Clashing directness   Clashing unipolar nar-
            with lightness.   rowing with a looping
                                   reversal in design.

      ii. Between Subsystems

          Examples: Examples:
            Affine even level   Affine bipolar widen-
            of tension and   ing with bipolar leng-
            strength.   thening.
            Clashing flexibility   Clashing-looping-de-
            with acceleration.   sign with descending.

   b) Specific Affinity or Specific Clashing Using
      Homogeneous 18) Qualities Through the Selection
      of Consonant and Dissonant Attributes and Elements

          Examples: Examples:
            Consonant high in-   Consonant shortening
            tensity of tension   with moving downward
            with vehemence or   or descending.
            strength.
            Dissonant even level   Dissonant angular re-
            of tension with flex- versal in design with
            ibility or indirect-   going forward or ad-
            ness.   vancing.

16) Note that there are three shape-flow subsystems
    which correspond to one tension-flow subsystem
    while shaping in directions corresponds to pre-
    cursors of effort and shaping in planes to efforts.

17) Heterogeneous qualities are represented on non-cor-
    responding lines of diagrams in the same subsystem
    or in different subsystems.

18) Homogeneous qualities are represented on correspond-
    ing lines of diagrams in the vertical affinity and
    horizontal affinity.

2.

HORIZONTAL AFFINITIES AND CLASHING
BETWEEN THE TWO MOVEMENT SYSTEMS

I. <u>Movement System: Effort</u>   II. <u>Movement System: Shape</u>
Composed of the Subsystems: Composed of the Subsystems:
Tension-Flow Attributes;   Shape-Flow (Bipolar, Uni-
                             polar and Design) Attributes;
Precursors of Effort;   Shaping in Directions;
Effort Elements.   Shaping in Planes Elements.

a) <u>General Affinity or Clashing between "Fighting"
and "Closed-Shaped" or between "Indulging" and
"Open-Shaped" Heterogeneous Attributes and Elements.</u>

  i) Within corresponding subsystems (tension
     and shape-flow, precursors of effort and
     shaping in directions, effort and shaping
     in planes).
     Examples: Affine low intensity of tension
               and widening;
               Clashing strength and advancing.

  ii) Between non-corresponding subsystems.
      Examples: Affine low intensity of tension
                and spreading;
                Clashing gentleness and advanc-
                ing.

b) <u>Specific Affinity or Clashing between Corresponding
Subsystems, Using Homogeneous Qualities Through the
Selection of Matching or Mismatching Attributes and
Elements</u>

     Examples: Matching of high intensity with
               either bipolar or unipolar
               shortening and/or high amplitudes
               in design.
               Mismatching of gradual ascent of
               tension with either bipolar or
               unipolar hollowing and/or angular
               reversals in design.
               Matching of flexibility with mov-
               ing sideways.
               Mismatching of gentleness with
               moving downward.
               Matching of directness with en-
               closing.
               Mismatching of acceleration with
               advancing.

PROFILE - GLENDA

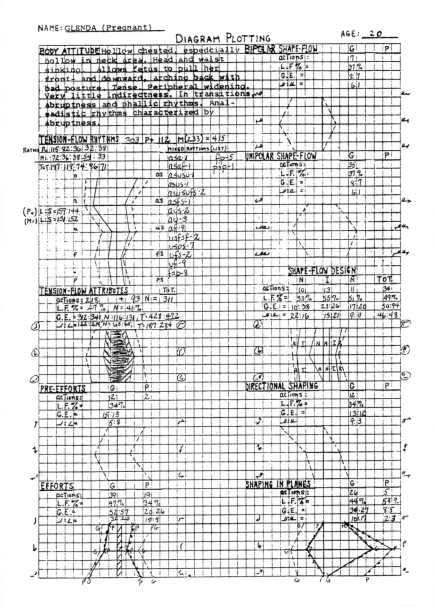

NAME: GLENDA (Pregnant)   AGE: 20

DIAGRAM PLOTTING

BODY ATTITUDE: Hollow chested, espedcially hollow in neck area. Head and waist sinking. Allows fetus to pull her front- and downward, arching back with bad posture. Tense. Peripheral widening. Very little indirectness. In transitions abruptness and phallic rhythms. Anal-sadistic rhythms characterized by abruptness.

BIPOLAR SHAPE-FLOW	G	P
actions:	17	
L.F.% =	31%	
G.E. =	3:7	
↲:↳ =	6:1	

TENSION-FLOW RHYTHMS 303 P+ 112 M(233) = 415

Ratios Pu: 115:92:36:32:38

Mi: 72:36:38:54: 33

Tot:187:118:74:86:71

MIXED RHYTHMS (LIST)

asa-1   fp-5
asaf-1   pspr-1
ois asusu-1
asus-1
asusufs-2
as asfs-1
aus-2
au-3
us af-9
usfsf-2
usps-7
fis ufs-2
uf-9
ps up-8

(Pu) L:S=159:144
(Mi) L:S=151:152

UNIPOLAR SHAPE-FLOW	G	P
actions:	35	
L.F.%:	37%	
G.E. =	8:7	
↲:↳ =	6:1	

TENSION-FLOW ATTRIBUTES

actions: 218   +: 93 N = 311
L.F.% = 27%   N = 41%
G.E. = 312:341 N:116:131, T: 428:472
↲:↳=122:214 N=65:65, T: 187:284

SHAPE-FLOW DESIGN	N	I	R	TOT.
actions:	10	13	11	34
L.F.% =	33%	55%	51%	49%
G.E. =	10:38	23:26	17:20	50:94
↲:↳ =	22:16	15:21	9:11	46:48

PRE-EFFORTS	G	P
actions:	121	2
L.F.% =	34%	
G.E. =	15:13	
↲:↳ =	5:8	

DIRECTIONAL SHAPING	G	P
actions:	12	
L.F.% =	34%	
G.E. =	13:12	
↲:↳ =	9:3	

EFFORTS	G	P
actions:	391	191
L.F.% =	47%	34%
G.E. =	52:57	26:26
↲:↳ =	32:20	19:8

SHAPING IN PLANES	G	P
actions:	26	5
L.F.% =	44%	54%
G.E. =	34:27	8:5
↲:↳ =	10:17	2:3

129

PROFILE - CHARLIE

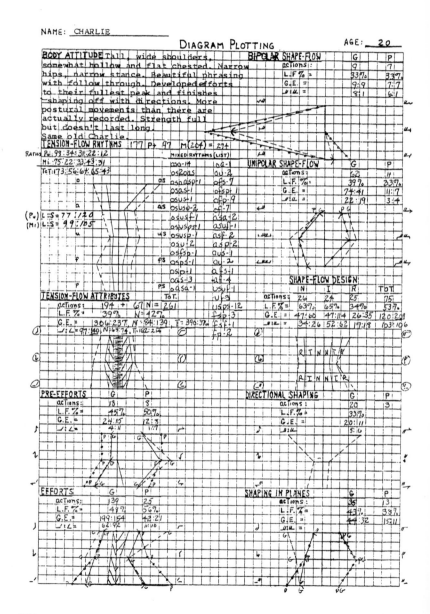

NAME: CHARLIE

DIAGRAM PLOTTING

AGE: 20

BODY ATTITUDE: Tall, wide shoulders, somewhat hollow and flat chested. Narrow hips, narrow stance. Beautiful phrasing with follow through. Developed efforts to their fullest peak and finishes shaping off with directions. More postural movements than there are actually recorded. Strength full but doesn't last long. Same old Charlie.

PROFILE - NANCY

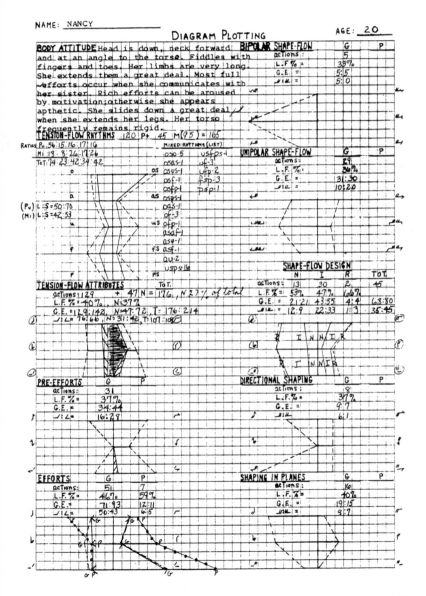

GLOSSARY

ACTION: A movement in which we can discern one, two or three attributes or elements in a given motion factor: as a tension-flow action, an effort action, a shaping action.

ACTION-DRIVE*: An action, composed of three effort elements, with an inner tendency (drive, in Laban's terms) to do something practical that has a concrete impact on the environment. In such an action, the flow element is latent. Synonyms: Full effort, complete effort.

ACTIVE: A quality of a motion-factor whose goal is to institute changes in the environment (Kestenberg & Marcus, 1979). See Activity & Passive.

ACTIVITY: An ongoing process of variations in which active and passive modes or aims alternate. One of the aims can predominate over the other. See Active and Passive.

AFFINITY: A good fit between patterns. Its opposite is clashing. We distinguish between vertical and horizontal affinity.

Vertical affinity pertains to related patterns in the two systems: 1) Tension-flow-effort and 2) Shape-flow-shaping.

Harmony in 1 reflects a compatibility between affects, defenses and coping mechanisms. Harmony in 2 reflects a compatibility between self-feelings (comfort-discomfort, attraction-repulsion), the styles and the modes of approaching and relating to people. There is a general and a specific vertical affinity.

General affinity in 1 is based on the compatibility of either all qualities subsumed under the heading "fighting" or all qualities subsumed under the heading "indulging". Angry feelings are affine with aggressive

---

All definitions of effort and shaping elements, their consonance and their dissonance, matching and mismatching, merging and clashing in postures and gestures, and their use in communication, presentation and operation are adapted from and modified after Laban (1947, 1960), Lamb (1961, 1065), Lamb & Turner (1969) and Ramsden (1973). The psychological correlations and interpretations are entirely our own.

The terms which were not used in the text are marked with an asterisk. They are included here to make the glossary more comprehensive to those familiar with Laban's original interpretations of effort (1960).

Affinity cont. Vertical affinity cont.

defenses and with aggressive modes of coping. Pleasant feelings are affine with peaceable defenses and with accommodating types of coping with the environment.

General affinity in 2 is based on the compatibility of "closed-shaped" and "open-shaped" qualities, respectively. Discomfort is affine with repulsion, with an abrasive style, with barring access to one's body and protectiveness. Comfort is affine with attraction, a smooth style, opening access to one's body and exposure to contact.

Specific vertical affinity is based on the compatibility of genetically related consonant patterns. In system 1, specific affects (such as being unruffled), specific defenses (such as isolation) and specific coping mechanisms (such as precision) are consonant. In system 2, specific self-feelings (such as generosity and seeking stimuli), specific styles (such as spiraling), specific defenses (such as exposing access to the upper part of the body) and specific forms of relating (such as opening up contact to groups of people) are consonant. For a listing of consonant qualities see Consonance.

Horizontal affinity pertains to related patterns of the two systems: 1. Tension-flow-effort and 2. Shape-flow-shaping.

Harmony between 1 and 2 reflects the compatibility:
a) between feelings in the safety-danger area (ease and anxiety) and self-feelings (comfort-discomfort and attraction-repulsion) as well as styles or manners and
b) between defenses against drives or affects and defenses against objects and
c) between coping with the environment and coping with objects.

General affinity pertains to the compatibility of "fighting" with "close-shaped" and of "indulging" with "open-shaped" motions. Anger is affine with constriction, shrinking away from, with angularity, with looking down and with retreating. Pleasant feelings are affine with generosity, attraction, smoothness, open-mindedness and· inviting of contact.

Specific horizontal affinity is based on the compatibility of genetically related matching patterns. Low intensity and lengthening or using small amplitudes which become dominant as matched sets at the same developmental stage are specifically affine. For a listing of matched patterns in 1 and 2 see Matching.

AGGRESSION: All impulses and activities which serve severing, disconnecting and breaking up. This definition is modelled after Freud's (1920) description of the aims of the death instinct, which turns into agression when directed outward. See Aggressive, erotic, libido, indulgence and indulging.

AGGRESSIVE: A quality of aggression which may pertain to affects, defenses and coping mechanisms. Aggressive affects are connected with displeasure, aggressive defense mechanisms aim at suppressing drives and aggressive coping with reality aims at displacing, contending and hurrying. See "Fighting" under effort.

ALIGNMENT*: Pertains to the way the body fits into spatial planes. Standing erect or lying down and fitting the body as closely as possible to the door, wall or floor respectively constitutes vertical alignment in the "door plane." Leaning forward or backward and balancing with one's arms in a suspended position constitutes horizontal alignment in the "table-plane." Reducing movement to the right and to the left as much as possible and making the body appear like an arrow constitutes sagittal alignment in the "wheel-plane".

ASYMMETRIC: See Shape-Flow.

ATTRIBUTES: Qualities of tension-flow and shape-flow which are called intensity factors and dimensional factors, respectively. See tension-flow and shape-flow.

AWAKE*: See efforts, incomplete.

BALANCE: A sufficient backing of specific patterns in the two movement systems. See Imbalance and Matching.

BASIC EFFORTS: See Efforts.

BODY ATTITUDE : Connotes all that can be seen in rest and movement and that can be described without notation. It refers to preferred shapes and alignments in planes, to the use of body parts together and separately and in relation to one another, to areas of high tension or neutral flow, and to all preferred patterns and phrases for which there is readiness at rest and which can be easily discerned during movement.

BODY SHAPE: Defined by the dimensions of the body (wide-narrow, long-short, bulging-hollow) and their relative size.

BOUND FLOW: See Flow.

BULGING: See Shape-flow.

CENTRALIZATION: A method of flow regulation in which all parts of the body, simultaneously or successively, undergo flow changes in consonance with a localized functional activity. For instance, the whole body of a drummer contributes to the tension-flow attributes of the arms. Centralization is a prototype of postural movements in efforts and shaping.

CHANNELING: See precursors of effort.

CLASHING: Connotes patterns which do not fit well together, for instance, low intensity and strength, directness and ascending or an acceleration in gesture followed by deceleration in posture. There is clashing within and between subsystems. There is general and specific clashing. Clashing is an expression of disharmony or conflict. See affinity, consonance, matching and gesture.

CLOSE-SHAPED: Pertains to shape-flow and shaping patterns which reduce contact with the environment. Closed shapes are concave shapes of the body or concave shapes created n space by close-shaped attributes or elements, respectively.

COMMUNICATION: See Matching.

CONFLICT: An opposition between two tendencies in the psyche. Conflicts can be intersystenic or intrasystemic (Hartmann, 1939). The former pertain to opposition between functions of the id and the ego or the id-ego and the superego; the latter pertain to opposition of functions within one psychic agency such as id, ego or superego. External conflicts pertain to opposition to external objects; internal conflicts pertain to opposition within the psyche and internalized conflicts pertain to those which had been transformed from external conflicts through internalization. Clashing, dissonance and mismatching of patterns connote conflicts.

CONSONANCE AND DISSONANCE: Affinity or clashing between genetically related patterns in the two systems of movement. Genetic relatedness pertains to specific antecedents of effort elements in system 1 and to specific antecedents of shaping elements in system 2.

Consonant Patterns in System 1.	Dissonant Patterns in System 1.
Even level of tension-channeling	Even level of tension-flexibility
Even level of tension-directness	Even level of tension-indirectness
Channeling-directness	Channeling-indirectness
Flow adjustment-flexibility	Flow adjustment-channeling
Flow adjustment-indirectness	Flow adjustment-directness
Flexibility-indirectness	Flexibility-directness
High intensity of tension-strength	High intensity-gentleness
High intensity " " -vehemence	High intensity-lightness
Vehemence-strength	Vehemence-lightness
Low intensity of tension-gentleness	Low intensity-vehemence
Low intensity " " -lightness	Low intensity-strength
Gentleness-lightness	Gentleness-strength
Abruptness-suddenness	Abruptness-hesitation
Abruptness-acceleration	Abruptness-deceleration
Suddenness-acceleration	Suddenness-deceleration
Graduality-hesitation	Graduality-Suddenness
Graduality-deceleration	Graduality-acceleration
Hesitation-deceleration	Hesitation-acceleration

Consonance and Dissonance cont.

Consonant Patterns in System 2	Dissonant Patterns in System 2
Bipolar or unipolar	Bipolar or unipolar
Narrowing-linear design	Narrowing-looping design
Narrowing-direction across	Narrowing-direction sideways
Narrowing-enclosing	Narrowing-spreading
Linear design-direction across	Linear design-direction sideways
Linear design-enclosing	Linear design-spreading
Direction across-enclosing	Direction across-spreading
Bipolar or unipolar	Bipolar or unipolar
Widening-looping design	Widening-linear design
Widening-direction sideways	Widening-direction across
Looping design-direction sideways	Looping design-direction across
Looping design-spreading	Looping design-enclosing
Direction sideways-spreading	Direction sideways-enclosing
Bipolar or unipolar	Bipolar or unipolar
Lengthening-small amplitude	Lengthening-large amplitude
Lengthening-direction upward	Lengthening-direction downward
Small amplitude-direction upward	Small amplitude-direction downward
Small amplitude-ascending	Small amplitude-descending
Direction upward-ascending	Direction upward-descending
Bipolar or unipolar	Bipolar or unipolar
Shortening-large amplitude	Shortening-small amplitude
Shortening-direction downward	Shortening-direction upward
Large amplitude-direction downward	Large amplitude-direction upward
Large amplitude-descending	Large amplitude-direction upward
Direction downward-descending	Direction downward-ascending
Bipolar or unipolar	Bipolar or unipolar
Hollowing-angular design	Hollowing-rounded design
Hollowing-direction backward	Hollowing-direction forward
Angular design-direction backward	Angular design-direction forward
Angular design-retreating	Angular design-advancing
Direction backward-retreating	Direction backward-advancing
Bipolar or unipolar	Bipolar or unipolar
Bulging-rounded design	Bulging-angular design
Bulging-direction forward	Bulging-direction backward
Rounded design-direction forward	Rounded design-direction backward
Rounded design-advancing	Rounded design-retreating
Direction forward-advancing	Direction forward-retreating

It should be noted that in unipolar shape-flow, lengthening can be cephalad or caudad (in the first instance it is consonant as above, in the second instance it is consonant with large amplitudes and with downward direction and descending); shortening can be caudad or cephalad (in the first instance it is consonant as above, in the second instance it is consonant with small amplitudes, and with upward direction and ascending); bulging can occur anteriorly or posteriorly (in the first instance it is consonant as above, in the second instance it is consonant with an angular design, backward direction and retreating); hollowing can occur posteriorly or anteriorly (in the first instance it is consonant as above, in the second instance it is consonant with rounded design, with a forward direction and advancing).

Glossary

CONTENDING: See effort.
DABBING*: See effort, basic.
DESIGN: See shape-flow design.
DIMENSIONS: See Shape-flow.
DIRECTIONS: See shaping of space in directions.
DISSONANCE: See consonance and dissonance.
DREAM-LIKE*: See efforts, incomplete.
EFFORT: A motion-factor which expresses changes in our
    attitude towards space, weight and time. Efforts
    serve the ego's adaptive functions and are used by
    the ego to mediate between drive expressions and ex-
    ternal reality. Effort elements mature gradually.
    Their forerunners are tension flow-attributes and
    elements of precursors of effort.

Laban (1960) distinguishes between the mechanical aspect of the effort, the movement sensation which accom-
panies it and the mental attitude which originates it.
The basic polarities of effort are:
1) "Fighting" (contending, resisting, withholding)
    elements which actively deal with space, weight and
    time. We assume that they are aggressive types of
    adaptation.
2) "Indulging" (yielding, enduring, accepting) elements
    which deal with space, weight and time passively.
    We assume that they belong to the life-sustaining
    tendencies in adaptation.
The "Fighting" elements are:
    a) Direct approach to space which divides space into
        geometric figures and is used in precise, blunt,
        and clear-cut motions.
    b) Strong action which counteracts gravity and conten
        with weight. It is used in determined, firm, pres
        suring, authoritative motions.
    c) Accelerating action which resists the passage of
        time and is used in decisive, timely and effective
        motions.
The "Indulging" elements are:
    a) Indirect approach to space which indulges in free
        forms and is used in wavy, pliant, intricate motic
    b) Light action which responds with buoyance to grav:
        and with "levity" to weight. It is used in fine
        touch, light pressure, decreasing pressure and in
        springy motions.
    c) Decelerating action which sustains the passage of
        time and is used in slowing down, luxuriating, lan
        guid motions.
Since Laban subsumed under the heading "effort" also the
qualities of motion which we classify as tension-flow
attributes and precursors of effort, he and his students
used various terms for effort elements. Having subdivie
effort into three subsystems we adhere strictly to our
terminology (See also tension-flow and precursors of
effort). A brief list of terms, other than those we use

Effort cont.

follows. Flexible is used for indirect, firm for strong, gentle for light, quick or sudden for accelerating and sustained for decelerating. We follow Lamb's terms for time efforts: "accelerating" and "decelerating". He speaks of directing and indirecting while we prefer to speak of a direct or indirect approach to space. He speaks of increasing and decreasing pressure while we prefer to speak of strength dealing with or counteracting gravity and lightness dealing with or responding to gravity.

Approaching Space Directly or Indirectly is used in the service of Attention, investigation and forethought.

Dealing with Gravity through Strong or Light effort elements is used in the service of Intention, determination and evaluation.

Coping with Time by Accelerating or Decelerating is used in the service of Decision, conclusion and effectiveness.

Laban referred to Flow as an Effort Element. He stated that in an Action-Drive*, consisting of three effort elements, the flow factor is dormant. He enumerated three other "drives*" in which flow replaced an effort element:

Passion-Drive*: in which space is replaced by flow, so that bodily actions become particularly expressive of emotion.

Vision-Drive*: in which weight is replaced by flow and thus bodily import is reduced.

Spell-Drive*: in which time is replaced by flow and the movement radiates a quality of fascination.

It seems that the so-called Action-Drive is synonymous with full or basic* efforts, in which three effort elements are represented. Full effort is sometimes referred to as having four elements of motion, space, weight, time and flow. Laban (1960) assigns feelings to flow changes.

Basic Effort Actions are:
Punching (direct, strong and accelerating), Floating (indirect, light and decelerating), Dabbing (direct, light and accelerating), Pressing (direct, strong and decelerating), Slashing (indirect, strong and accelerating), Wringing (indirect, strong and decelerating), Flicking (indirect, light and accelerating) and Gliding (direct, light and decelerating).

Incomplete* effort actions contain two effort elements. They are said to be expressive of Inner Attitudes*, such as these:

Stable attitudes in actions composed of space and weight elements (steady, balanced).

Near* attitudes in actions composed of weight and time elements (earthy, rhythmic).

Awake* attitudes in actions composed of space and time
elements (alert).

Dreamlike* or dreamy attitudes in actions composed of
weight and flow elements (referring to bodily
feelings and hazy fantasies).

Mobile attitudes in actions composed of time and flow
elements (mobilizing, getting on, progressing).

Remote* attitudes in actions composed of space and
flow elements (pensive, visualizing, projecting
outward).

Our notation of effort elements pertains to variations
(See also Lamb, 1961). For instance strength is notated
when it appears, not when it persists. If it is noted
again, it indicates that strength had subsided and appeared again. Notations in which effort elements are
noted as long as they persist connote states of adapt-
edness rather than adaptation.

EGO: In psychoanalytic terminology, a psychic structure
which mediates between the id (a representative of
bodily needs) and external reality. It comprises sets
of functions which can be divided into defensive and
coping. These functions operate on conscious, pre-
conscious or unconscious levels. The ego, in contrast
to the id, symbolizes reasonableness; it monitors fantasy in accordance with the reality principle. The ego
develops gradually, forming from the id under the influence of reality and from an autonomous apparatus
(Hartmann, 1939). The superego develops out of the ego,
becoming a separate psychic agency which supervises,
punishes and shames the ego. The term "ego" was and
still is sometimes used in lieu of the term "self".
See also id, reality, self and superego .

ELEMENTS: Refer to qualities of flow (free or bound,
growing or shrinking) and to qualities of all patterns
except those of tension- and shape-flow which are
called attributes.

EROTIC: Erotic or sexual drives are (according to Freud,
1920) expressions of a life sustaining instinct, Eros,
whose aim is to bind, combine and connect. The energy
with which the erotic drives are said to operate is
called libido. We refer to life-sustaining tendencies
as "indulging", but we retain the term "libidinal" to
classify tension-flow rhythms. The polarity of Eros
is Thanatos, the death instinct. See also aggression,
indulging, libido, rhythms of tension-flow.

FIGHTING: See effort.

FLEXIBLE: See precursors of effort.

FLICKING*: See efforts, basic.

FLOW: Refers to the range of continuity and discontinuity in movement and to freedom of movement and restraint. Laban (1960) referred to the former as flux. Free, fluid movement cannot be easily stopped at will; bound, hampered movement can be stopped at any point. We distinguish between a flow of tension and a flow of shape.

FLOW OF EFFORT: Refers to the fluency or constraint with which efforts proceed. Laban looked upon flow as an effort element. He pointed out that in free flow agonistic muscles have a free range of movement and in bound flow there is simultaneous contraction of antagonists. In agreement with Lamb (1961) we do not think of flow as an effort. Flow is a carrier of feeling and is thus of a different category than efforts which serve adaptation to external reality.

FLOW OF TENSION: Pertains to the sequence of fluency and restraint in muscles during movement and rest. It depends on the elasticity of tissue and is controlled by the gamma nervous system. The basic elements of tension-flow are free and bound flow. The attributes of tension-flow, referred to as intensity factors are: even or adjusted level of tension, high and low intensity, abrupt or gradual increase and decrease of tension. See also tension-flow.

FLOW REGULATION: Organizes changes in shape-flow and tension-flow in the service of functions. It is one of the first motion factors which comes under the control of the early ego. Immobilization, localization of shape- and tension-changes, melody of movement, mobilization, modification of rhythm, modulation of tension-flow, phrasing of rhythmic patterns, redistribution of shape-flow and tension-flow in various parts of the body, the selection of their elements and attributes and their sequencing, full and partial stabilization of shape and tension, as well as subordination of flow to effort and shaping respectively, are all methods of flow regulation. These are explained under their respective headings.

FLOW OF SHAPE: Pertains to the sequence of expansion and constriction of body-shape (Lamb, 1961). It depends on the plasticity of tissue and it is related to the flow of tension. The basic elements of shape-flow are growing and shrinking. The attributes of shape-flow referred to as dimensional factors are: narrowing and widening, shortening and lengthening, hollowing and bulging. For differences in bipolar and unipolar shape-flow and in shape-flow design see Shape-Flow-Design.

FLUX: See flow.

FREE FLOW: See flow.

Glossary

FULL EFFORT*: An action in which there are three effort
elements; for instance, directness, strength, and
acceleration used simultaneously in punching. It may
also contain bound or free flow. See also action,
drive and effort, basic.

FULL SHAPE*: An action in which there are three shaping
elements; for instance, spreading, ascending and advancing used simultaneously to open up space to the
fullest degree. It may also contain growing or shrinking.

GAIN-EXPENSE: a ratio between attributes of tension-flow
and the sum total of changes in bound and free flow; a
ratio between attirbutes of shape-flow and the sum
total of growing and shrinking; a ratio between elements of precursors of effort or effort and the sum
total of free and bound flow, which accompanied these
patterns respectively; a ratio between attributes of
shape-flow-design and the sum total of centripetal and
centrifugal movement; the ratio between shaping in
directions or shaping in planes and the sum total of
the growing and shrinking which accompanied these
patterns respectively.

   The gain expense ratio indicates the degree to
which there is a gain in attributes or elements over
the expense through simple fluctuations in flow. If
the former is high, it signifies a high degree of
control over emotions, and vice versa if the latter
is much higher than the former it indicates a high
degree of spontaneity and affective participation
with lesser control.

GATHERING*: See shaping.

GENTLE: See precursors of effort.

GESTURE: A movement in one part of the body which is performed in a certain pattern. For instance, we can see
low intensity in a gesture, or indirect effort in a
gesture. Gesture is contrasted with posture, in which
the same pattern is used by all parts of the body, to a
greater or lesser degree.

   Gestures are used to protect the organism from too
extreme exposure to danger. Effort and shaping, performed in a gesture which precedes a posture, are frequently seen in actions reflecting "thinking things
over on a trial basis". Effort and shaping performed
in gestures which follow a posture are frequently seen
in actions reflecting "testing the limits" of the almost completed action without exposing the whole body
of the mover to a hazard. When gestures and postures
use the same motion elements as they precede or succeed one another, we speak of gesture-posture or posture-gesture merging (Lamb, 1965).. When this occurs,
the aim of the actions remain the same, only the degree
of involvement has changed. Non-merging or clashing
between gestures and postures and vice versa implies
a change into a different or an opposite aim respec-

Gesture cont.

tively. Gesture-posture merging or vice versa, reflects harmony between the executive and the super-
vising mental structures (ego and superego). Frequent
clashes between gestures and postures suggest gaps and
conflicts between these structures. See also conflict
and postures.

GLIDING: See effort, basic.

HETEROGENEOUS: Pertains to patterns which are represented on different lines of the diagrams (see pp. 130-
132), for instance, even flow of tension (on line 1)
is heterogeneous-clashing to lightness and heterogeneous-affined to strength (both on line 2). Channeling
(on line 1) is heterogeneous-affined to descending and
heterogeneous-clashing to ascending (both on line 2).

HOLLOWING: See shape-flow.

HOMOGENEOUS: Pertains to patterns which are represented
on the same lines of the diagrams, for instance, even
flow of tension (on line 1) is homogeneous-affined to
directness and homogeneous-clashing to indirectness
(both on line 1); acceleration (on line 3) is homogeneous-clashing to bulging and homogeneous-affined
to hollowing (both on line 3).

HORIZONTAL: See shaping in planes.

ID: In psychoanalytic terminology a psychic structure
in which bodily needs are expressed in drives. All of
the psychic functions of the id are unconscious. The
ego differentiates from the id under the impact of
reality. Freud spoke of the id-ego as originally one.
In the text, the term "id-ego" refers to the two structures combined and differentiated from the superego.

IMBALANCE: Pertains to a relationship between effort and
shaping (and other related subsystems) in which there
is neither matching nor mismatching between related
patterns, but one is abundant while the other is absent
or scanty. For instance acceleration may be in abundance while there is little retreating and at the same
time deceleration and advancing are fully matched.
Effort without a related shaping pattern, shaping without a related effort pattern are at the core of an
imbalance in the ego.

IMMOBILIZATION: A mechanism of flow-regulation, most frequently achieved by the introduction of bound flow.

INCOMPLETE*effort: Pertains to actions performed with
two effort elements. They express inner attitudes
(Laban, 1960). See effort, incomplete.

INDULGING: See effort.

INTENSITY: Refers to the intensity of tension. See tension-flow.

INTERSYSTEMIC: Pertains to conflict between one psychic
structure and another, as between id and ego or ego
and superego (Hartmann, 1939).

Glossary

INTRASYSTEMIC: Pertains to conflicts within a psychic
structure--in the id, in the ego or in the superego.
See system.

LENGTHENING: See shape-flow.

LIBIDINAL: In psychoanalysis, the adjective derived from
libido, defined as the energy with which Eros, the
life-sustaining instinct or sexual drives operate.
Used here as a term for rhythms, suitable for this type
of drive discharge, it can be defined in movement as a
type of rhythm in which "indulging" tension-flow attributes predominate.

LIBIDO: Freud's term for the energy of sexual or erotic
drives or of the life-instinct (1920). Within this
framework, aggressive energy belongs to the aggressive
drives and to the death instinct.

LOAD-FACTOR: Pertains to the complexity with which a
movement is performed. In each subsystem (with the
exception of rhythms of tension-flow) one can move in
one only, two or three ways in one action. For instance, one can use high intensity, adjustment of
tension-level and graduality, either singly or in a
combination. Obviously one cannot use high and low
intensity at the same time. Another example is the
use of direct, strong and decelerating effort elements,
either singly or in combination of two or three elements. The more attributes or elements used in a
single action, the higher the load-factor and the more
complex the action. If all actions are performed with
three elements, the L-F on top of the profile diagram
is 100%; if they all contain only one element, the
L-F on top of the profile diagram is 33%. Ordinarily
there are variations in the loading of individual actions and the L-F on top of each diagram is a composite
of all action-loadings.

LOCALIZATION: A mechanism of flow regulation which initiates and maintains zone-specific patterns of flow
changes in functionally related parts of the body.
Thus, a sucking rhythm becomes dominant in the mouth
region or a rhythm appropriate to grasping becomes dominant in the hand. Localization is a prototype for
moving in gestures.

MATCHING: Of patterns is based on their affinity. Matching is a specific inter-system affinity between the
two main movement systems. It refers to the mechanisms
of pairing of
1) specific attributes of tension-flow with corresponding homogeneous attributes of bipolar and unipolar
shape-flow and shape-flow-design,
2) specific precursors of effort with corresponding
homogeneous shaping in directions, and
3) specific effort elements with corresponding
homogeneous shaping in planes.

Matching cont.

1.

Matched patterns of tension- and shape-flow and shape-flow-design are based on the polarities of:

Tension-flow attributes, which are forerunners of "fighting" efforts, and shape-flow attributes, which are forerunners of shaping to restrict contact with the environment (= "closed-shapes"); Tension-flow attributes, which are forerunners of "indulging" efforts, and shape-flow attributes which are forerunners of shaping to promote contact with the environment (= "open-shapes").

Tension	Shape	Design
Bound Flow	Shrinking	Centripetal
Fighting tension-flow attributes:	Closed-shape bipolar & unipolar shape-flow attributes	Forbidding design attributes
even level	Narrowing - medial	linear pathways
high intensity	shortening - caudal	large amplitudes
abrupt change	hollowing - posterior	angular reversals

Tension	Shape	Design
Free flow	Growing	Centrifugal
Indulging tension-flow attributes	Open shape bipolar and unipolar shape-flow attributes	Permissive design attributes
adjustment of level	widening - lateral	loops or waves
low intensity	lengthening- cephalad	small amplitudes
gradual changes	bulging - frontal	rounded reversals

Matching between tension-flow and bipolar shape-flow expresses harmony between feelings of danger or safety and corresponding feelings of discomfort and comfort. Matching between tension-flow and unipolar shape-flow expresses harmony between feelings of danger and safety and feelings of repulsion and attraction. Matching between tension-flow and shape flow-design expresses harmony between feelings of danger and safety and crude, forbidding or fine permissive forms of relating. Mismatching of these patterns expresses clashes between the specific categories of feelings.

2.

Matched or affined elements of precursors of effort and shaping in directions are based on the affined polarities of:

"fighting" and restricting the boundaries of spatial areas versus

"indulging" and extending the boundaries of spatial areas.

Fighting elements	Restricting elements
Precursors of effort	Shaping in directions
channeling	moving across the body
vehemence	moving downward
suddenness	moving backward

Indulging elements	Extending elements
Precursors of effort	Shaping in directions
flexibility	moving sideways
gentleness	moving upward
hesitation	moving forward

Matching of precursors of effort and shaping in directions expresses harmony between motor expressions of modes of learning or defense mechanisms against drives and those related to localized objects. Mismatching of these patterns reveals clashes and conflicts between these attitudes. For instance, learning to play basketball, one encounters difficulties when trying to throw the ball upwards with vehemence. Or, the defense gets distorted when channeling-- a motor form of isolation-- is attempted while pointing sideways, extending rather than restricting spatial boundaries.

3.

Matched or affined elements of effort and shaping in planes are based on the polarities of:

"fighting" and "closed shapes"; and

"indulging" and "open shapes".

Fighting	Closing off Space
Effort	Shaping in Planes
directness	enclosing
strength	descending
acceleration	retreating

Indulging	Opening up Space
Effort	Shaping in Planes
indirectness	spreading
lightness	ascending
deceleration	advancing

Matching of effort and shaping elements reveals harmony between adaptation to reality and relationships to people. Mismatching of these patterns expresses conflicts in this area.

The spheres of conflict-free communication, presentation and operation (Lamb & Turner, 1969, Ramsden, 1973) can be defined by the matching of effort and shaping elements in the following way:

Communication is based on the functioning of attention which is supported by the exploration of objects in the spatial area which is being attended to. The mode of attention is revealed in the use of direct or indirect approaches to space. Exploration through enclosing and spreading of space structures attention. For optimal effects directness is combined with enclosing and indirectness with spreading. Conflicts in communication are based on the mismatching of these patterns so that direct effort elements are combined with spreading and indirect effort elements with enclosing. (Lamb, 1961, Ramsden, 1972).

Presentation is based on the presence of an in-

tention to confront someone with what one wants to
show or explain. The mode of intention is revealed
in the use of strength or lightness. It is structured by descending and ascending. For optimal effect, strength is combined with descending and lightness with ascending. Conflicts in presentation are
based on the mismatching of these patterns so that
strength is combined with ascending and lightness
with descending.

Operation is based on a good range of decision
making which is aided by the anticipation of the actions of others. The mode of decision-making is
revealed in the use of acceleration or deceleration.
It is structured by retreating and advancing. For
optimal effect, acceleration is combined with retreating and deceleration with advancing. Conflicts
in operation are expressed in the mismatching of
these patterns so that acceleration combines with
advancing and deceleration with retreating.

MELODY OF MOVEMENT: results from a flow regulation in
which flow-intensity is graduated in a selected
sequence.

MERGING: See gestures.

MIXED RHYTHMS: See rhythms of tension-flow.

MOBILE*: See efforts, incomplete.

MOBILIZATION: A combination of acceleration or deceleration with free or bound flow which, together, initiate
motion.

MODIFICATION OF RHYTHMS: A flow regulation in which one
rhythm is changed through attunement with another,
usually one that has been used by another person. An
infant who uses an "anal" rhythm for sucking may modify
it in order to conform to the "oral" rhythm with which
the milk is released from the breast. As a result he
may suck in an "oro-anal" rhythm.

MODULATION OF FLOW: A regulation by fine gradation of
intensities.

MOVEMENT DRIVE*: See effort, full.

NARROWING: See shape-flow.

NEAR*: See effort, incomplete.

NEUTRAL FLOW: Pertains to a loss of elasticity when it
concerns tension-flow; a loss of plasticity when it
concerns shape-flow. Examples of neutral tension are:
limpness, "Raggedy Ann" qualities, inertia, woodiness,
and catalepsy. Neutral flow is characteristic of
states of altered consciousness. Attributes of tension-flow, pre-effort and effort elements can all
proceed in neutral flow, as when inertia develops
abruptly, channeling turns into a daze or acceleration and limpness combine. Examples of neutral shape
are shapelessness, indescript sinking or appearing

Neutral Flow cont.

inflated like a balloon. In such states, body boundaries are either lost or diminished and there may be
a dissolution of the body image. Dimensional changes
in the shape of the body at such times are not the
result of shape-flow regulation, but are rather mechanical changes due to external circumstances. For
instance, seated in a large chair, the person who is
in neutral shape-flow will automatically fill the
chair because there is room. A certain degree of
neutral flow is used by everyone, depending on the
state of the body. It is particularly noticeable
during tiredness and illness.

NON-MERGING: See gestures.

OBJECT: In psychoanalytic terminology, the word "object"
refers to an internal representation of a person.

OPEN-SHAPES: See shape-flow, shaping in planes and matching.

PASSION*: See effort, drives.

PASSIVE: A quality of a motion-factor whose goal is to
accommodate to the external reality. See active,
activity.

PHRASING: The sequential grouping of motion factors to
form distinct phrases of movement. Phrasing can be accomplished by a flow regulation which selects sequences
of rhythms and patterns or by a sequential distribution
of effort and shaping, or by similar means. Phrasing
can be uni-phasic or multiphasic. A typical phrasing
consists of 1) an introduction, 2) a main theme of
action, and 3) its resolution or ending--which may at
the same time be a transition to the next phrase.

PLANES OF SPACE: See shaping in planes.

POSTURES: Do not pertain to static positions of the body
but to movement in which the whole body participates in
in one or more identical patterns. A prototype of postural movements is the centralization of flow. We can
distinguish global postures from integrated postures.

In global postures, the whole body uses the same patterns in the same way, as in jumping up and down or
stomping with strength. In integrated postures, all
parts of the body cooperate in the support of a pattern, without being equally involved, for example, in
ascending with lightness, this pattern is more clearly
developed in the upper than in the lower part of the
body and at least one leg is used for support. Global
postures are usually symmetrical and lead to changes
of position. Integrated postures are usually asymmetrical and they need not lead to changes of position.
Postural movements are used in actions in which the
mover is totally involved. This implies wholehearted-
ness and a lack of reservation, based on the harmonious
participation of all psychic agencies including the

superego. Shaping and efforts are noted in gestures of young children. Postural changes in these patterns develop from global to highly integrated total body participation. <u>Global postures</u> are seen regularly, and <u>integrated postural</u> movements begin to appear with some frequency in latency. <u>Merging</u> gestures into postures and vice versa begins in adolescence and becomes the most important characteristic of adult phrases of movement. See also gestures.

PRECURSORS OF EFFORT: Patterns which develop from modes of tension-flow-regulation and precede and supplement efforts. Tension-flow regulates our internal environment by regulating feelings and drives. Efforts change our external environment through their control of space weight, and time. Precursors of effort attempt to change the external environment through their control of tension-flow attributes. Precursors of effort operate in immature actions, defensive actions and in learning, by using:

a) elements which serve active "fighting" behavior, and

b) elements which serve passive "indulging" behavio

a) Channelling actions (making use of even flow of tension) are precursors of direct effort actions.
    Vehement actions (making use of high intensity o tension) are precursors of strong effort actions.
    Sudden actions (making use of abrupt changes of tension) are precursors of accelerating effort actions.

b) Flexible actions (making use of adjustments of tension levels) are precursors of indirect effort actions.
    Gentle actions (making use of low intensity of tension) are precursors of light effort actions.
    Hesitating actions (making use of gradual changes of tension) are precursors of decelerating effort actions.

Note that Laban (1960) used the term "sudden" for accelerating effort, "flexible" for indirect efforts and "gentle" for light effort.
    See efforts.

PRESENTATION: See matching.
PRESSING*: See effort, basic.
PUNCHING: See effort, basic.
PURE RHYTHMS: See rhythms of tension-flow.
QUICK*: See effort.

REALITY: In psychoanalytic terminology, reality can be external or internal. The more subjective one's view of facts, the more we speak of internal reality. The representation of external reality in the ego corrects the products of fantasy which distort reality. In the terminology used here, external reality comprises the forces of nature governing life on our planet: space, gravity and time. Coping with external reality refers to the coping with these forces through effort.

REBOUND: A slight diminution of a quality immediately followed by its increase. Rebound is best known in sequences of jumping or tapping in which going up can be renewed by the interpolation of small excursions downward. This principle is applied to any quality of movement. Rebound is a sign of resiliency.

REDISTRIBUTION OF FLOW: A flow regulation through which flow elements are changed in various parts of the body to initiate, maintain, change or stop a functional activity.

REMOTE*: See effort, incomplete.

RETIRING: See shaping in planes.

RETREATING: See shaping in planes.

RHYTHM: Periodic repetitions of variations in one or more quality. In regular rhythms, the intervals and the variations are consistently the same. Biological rhythms can be irregular in their intervals and variations.

RHYTHMS OF SHAPE-FLOW: Periodic alternations of growing and shrinking of body shape in simple rhythms, such as inhaling and exhaling. More complex rhythms are composed of repetitions of the dimensional attributes, such as narrowing or widening, shortening or lengthening and hollowing or bulging.

We distinguish rhythms of bipolar (symmetrical) shape-flow from those which repeat and alternate attributes of unipolar (asymmetrical) shape-flow. There are individual preferences for certain dimensional qualities in symmetric and asymmetrical shape-flow. For instance, some people breathe predominantly by lengthening and shortening, and others may bulge and widen while inhaling and hollow and narrow while exhaling. Turning to and away from stimuli--an example of asymmetrical shape-flow--takes on a rhythmic quality when the stimuli are rhythmic. Rhythms of asymmetrical shape-flow depend on the nature, frequency and intensity of the stimuli. Still, there are individual preferences for reacting to stimuli, as for instance a tendency to widen and narrow unilaterally without regard for the location from which the stimulus comes.

Because of its three-dimensional nature, shape-flow, unlike tension-flow, cannot be notated by a free-hand tracing on paper. By notating rhythms of shape-

flow in symbols, we do not have the opportunity to see
formal variations of individual rhythmic units. A
classification of these rhythms must await a better
method of notation.

RHYTHMS OF SHAPE-FLOW-DESIGN: Consist of a periodic
regular or irregular repetition of simple and complex
units of design with which we traverse space. Such a
unit may consist of a large centrifugal motion which
proceeds in a straight line, reverses roundly in a
series of centripetal waves, which may, for example,
bring a limb in touch with the face. Such a unit may
be repeated immediately or after an interval of time.
    Rhythms of shape-flow-design reflect styles of
interaction and customs of relating. See shape-flow-
design.

RHYTHMS OF TENSION-FLOW: Periodic alternations between
free and bound flow in simple rhythmic patterns (such
as sucking or snapping) and periodic alternations of
tension-flow attributes in complex rhythms. Rhythms
of tension-flow are responsible for the pleasure in
movement because they serve need-satisfaction in its
original and derived forms. For instance, "oral"
rhythms can be seen in the perioral region during
sucking, but they can be noted in pleasurable mouthing and speaking, in finger- and toe-play, in patting
and dabbing as well.
    We distinguish between:
        1) Pure rhythmic units which occur in various
        parts of the body, but are best suited for the
        achievement of satisfaction in specific zones
        of the body, and
        2) Mixed rhythmic units which result from a
        confluence of two or more pure rhythmic units,
        or from a modification by another rhythm, usu-
        ally in attunement with another person.
    We refer to rhythms as "libidinal" when their at-
tributes are predominantly of the "indulging" variety,
and are suitable for libidinal modes of drive discharge.
We refer to rhythms as "sadistic" when their attributes
are predominantly of the "fighting" variety, and they
are suitable for sadistic modes of drive discharge.
    We note the following pure rhythms as well as their
combinations:
a) Those which come into the service of libidinal drives:
    "Oral", a sucking type of rhythm;
    "Anal", a sphincter-like, twisting type of rhythm;
    "Urethral", a "walk-run" type of rhythm;
    "Inner-genital" ("feminine"), an undulating type of
    rhythm;
    "Phallic" ("outer-genital"), a jumping type of rhythm.

Rhythms of Tension-Flow cont.

 b) Those which come into the service of <u>sadistic</u> drives
   are:
   "Oral-sadistic", a snapping or biting type of rhythm;
   "Anal-sadistic", a straining type of rhythm;
   "Urethral-sadistic", a run-stop-go type of rhythm;
   "Inner-genital-sadistic", ("feminine"), a swaying
   type of rhythm;
   "Phallic-sadistic" ("outer-genital"), a leaping type
   of rhythm.
   Pure rhythms are more differentiated than mixed
rhythms. Both are available to the newborn. However,
phase-specific rhythms become more frequent and more
differentiated in appropriate developmental phases.
RISING*: See shaping.
<u>SADISTIC</u>: Pertains, in psychoanalytic usage, to a mixture
 of aggressive and libidinal drive components. Used here
 as a term for rhythms, suitable for a sadistic discharge,
 it can be defined in movement as a mixture of "fighting" and "indulging" tension-flow elements in which
 the former predominate. Examples are "oral-sadistic"
 biting or "phallic-sadistic" leaping. It has no con-
 notation of perversion nor does it connote an intent
 to hurt. See libidinal rhythms of tension-flow.
SAGITTAL: See Shaping in Planes.
<u>SCATTERING</u>*: See Shaping in Planes.
<u>SELECTION OF FLOW ELEMENTS AND THEIR ATTRIBUTES</u>: Flow
 regulation by planned selection of flow qualities in
 adaptation to reality; for instance, choosing even
 bound flow to reach a small object, or hollowing to
 initiate retreat. This type of regulation is a part-
 function of effort and shaping and their respective
 precursors.
<u>SELF</u>: In the terminology used here, "self" refers to the
 psychic representation of the individual. In its core,
 the "self" may consist of sensations and feelings of
 comfort or discomfort and other allied <u>self-feelings</u>.
 At first, the self and the object are not differentiated. With progressive ego development, the self differentiates from the object and their respective
 representations become permanent. See ego, shape-flow.
<u>SEQUENTIAL DISTRIBUTION OF FLOW ELEMENTS AND THEIR</u>
 <u>ATTRIBUTES</u>: Flow regulation by a selection of the sequence of patterns and rhythms.
<u>SHAPE-FLOW</u>: An apparatus which serves interaction with
 stimuli and objects in the environment. The basic elements of shape-flow are growing and shrinking of body
 shape. The shape of the body changes symmetrically
 and asymmetrically. We grow and shrink symmetrically
 as we inhale and exhale, using bipolar shape-flow. We
 grow and shrink asymmetrically when we respond to
 pleasant or noxious, localized stimuli using unipolar

shape-flow. The body-shape changes in one, two or three dimensions. The polarities of shape-flow are:
a) "Closed-shapes" which reduce the exposure of the body, including its inside, to the environment, and
b) "Open-shapes" which increase the exposure of the body, including its inside, to the environment.

"Closed-shaped" dimensional attributes of bipolar shape-flow are: shrinking by narrowing in width, shortening in length, and hollowing in depth, as seen in exhaling.

"Open-shaped" dimensional attributes of bipolar shape-flow are: growing by widening in width, lengthening in length, and bulging in depth, as seen in inhaling.

"Closed-shaped" dimensional attributes in unipolar shape-flow are: Shrinking towards the middle (medially), towards the bottom (caudad), towards the back (posteriorly); and shrinking towards the head (cephalad) and towards the front (anteriorly). Each of them protects a part of the body.

"Open-shaped" dimensional attributes in unipolar shape-flow are: growing towards the side (laterally), towards the head (cephalad), towards the front (frontally or anteriorly); and growing towards the bottom (caudad) and towards the back (posteriorly) of the body. Each of them exposes a part of the body.

Variations in shape are used to express changes in our affective relations to objects in the environment. Bipolar shape-flow expresses comfort and discomfort, as the organism reacts to air, temperature and similar environmental objects. Unipolar shape-flow is expressive of attraction and repulsion, as the organism reacts to salutory or noxious stimuli of a discrete nature.

Note that Laban (1960) and some of his pupils use the term "narrowing" for enclosing and the term "widening" for spreading. See flow of shape. For affine combinations of shape-flow attributes with shaping see consonance; for affine combinations with tension-flow attributes see matching.

SHAPE-FLOW DESIGN: An apparatus which permits the mover to traverse the space around him and create designs in space as he moves. Space can be divided into general space which is beyond reach and personal space, which is always with us.

In personal space movements are transacted in the:
"Near-Space", close to the body;
"Reach-Space", as far as one can reach;
"Intermediate Space", between the near-space and reach-space.

Shape-Flow Design cont.

The basic elements of spatial design in these areas
are:
Centripetal, directed towards the body, and
Centrifugal, directed outward, away from the body.
They proceed in:
Lines and curves or waves and loops
With high or low amplitude
By angular or rounded reversals of direction.
The apparatus of shape-flow-design is available
to the newborn, but most susceptible to cultural influences. It reflects styles of relationships and
manners, with linear, high amplitude and angular
movement conveying a crude or forbidding attitude,
and wavy, low amplitude and rounded movement conveying
a polite or permissive attitude.
SHAPING OF SPACE: Creating changes in the configuration
of space by introducing into it directional lines or
two or three dimensional shapes.
SHAPING OF SPACE IN DIRECTIONS: Divides space through
linear vectors. Directions are projections of body-
dimensions into space:
In the horizontal dimension width can be divided
into the directions "across the body" and "sideways".
In the vertical dimension length can be divided
into the directions "downward" and "upward".
In the sagittal dimension depth can be divided into
the directions "backward" and "forward".
Shaping in directions can be:
a) "Closed-shaped", barring access to the body by
linear boundaries.
b) "Open-shaped", delineating the outer limits of
access by linear boundaries.
a) Closed-shaped directions are: across the body,
downward and backward, all used for protection.
b) Open-shaped directions are sideways, upwards
and forward, all used for enlarging the limits of
exposure.
To localize distant objects, we reach within the
confines of our personal space and we point beyond our
reach-space into the general space, thus making it our
own. At the same time we use these directional movements for defenses against stimuli and objects by barring access to the body or by opening up boundaries for
appeasement. Both closed-shaped and open-shaped directional shaping are used for learning. Unipolar
shape-flow is a precursor of shaping in directions.
The former is intrinsic to the body-ego, the latter to
the ego proper. For affinity with other patterns of
the shape system see affinity, consonance and dissonance. For affinity with the effort-system, especially
homogeneous affinity, see matching.

SHAPING OF SPACE IN PLANES: Divides space into multi-dimensional shapes. The basic elements of shaping in planes are the two-dimensional "closing" and "opening" of space. When applied to shape-flow, "closed-shape" and "open-shape" refer to body-shape; when applied to shaping in directions they refer to restrictions and extensions of boundaries in the space around us; when applied to shaping in planes they refer to two or three-dimensional concave and convex shapes which our movements sculpt in space.

The "closing" and "opening" of multidimensional space occur in one, two or three of the following spatial planes:

The horizontal plane with its principal dimension "across-sideways" and its accessory dimension "backwards-forwards" (Laban's table-plane).

The vertical plane, with its principal dimension "downward-upward" and its accessory dimension "across-sideways" (Laban's door-plane).

The sagittal plane, with its principal dimension "backwards-forwards" and its accessory dimension "downward-upward" (Laban's wheel-plane).

Patterns which form closed (concave) shapes in these planes are:

Enclosing, descending and retreating.

Patterns which form open (convex) shapes in these planes are:

Spreading, ascending and advancing.

These elements are used singly or in combination with one another. The more elements there are in an action, the higher its load factor. Shaping of space in planes serves transactions with objects whose representation is multidimensional. The development of shaping from its immature to its mature forms goes hand in hand with the development of object-constancy (Kestenberg et al, 1971) and self-constancy, both evolving from identifications and complementarity of object- and self-shapes. All terms used by Lamb (1961) to define the function of shaping in planes refer to dealing with people or their internalized images:

Shaping in the horizontal plane is used for exploration.

Shaping in the vertical plane is used for confrontation.

Shaping in the sagittal plane is used for anticipation.

The more elements there are in one action, the higher its load-factor. That implies that in a highly loaded action, there is a greater chance for success in relating because several modes of approach are used.

It should be noted that Laban divided shaping elements into gathering and scattering, terms borrowed

Shaping of Space in Planes cont.

from the observation of reaping and sowing motions in dances. Lamb refers to the same distinction as con- cave and convex while we prefer to speak of closed- and open-shaped polarities of shaping. A common usage in effort-shape literature is to refer to spreading as widening, to enclosing as narrowing, to ascending as rising and to descending as sinking. Lamb (Ramsden, 1973) lately refers to retreating as retiring. See also consonance and matching.

SHORTENING: See shape-flow and flow of shape.

SINKING*: See shaping in planes.

SLASHING*: See effort, basic.

SLOW: Refers to a slow tempo, not to the slowing down in deceleration.

SPELL: See effort, drive.

SPREADING: See shaping in planes.

STABILIZATION: Flow-regulation that decreases the frequency of flow fluctuations. Complete stabilization leads to immobility in all parts of the body. Partial stabiliza- tion reduces flow-changes in certain parts of the body to prevent interference with localized motor discharge or gestures.

Stabilization can also refer to "becoming stable", that is, introducing combinations of space and weight efforts which, in contradistinction to combinations of time and flow, accentuate stability.

STABLE*: See effort, incomplete.

STATES: Periods of time in which certain patterns remain unchanged or vary insignificantly. When strength pre- vails for some time, we speak of a state of strength; when lightness prevails for some time, we speak of a state of lightness. Such "frozen"* patterns can become part of a person's body attitude. Using this concept one can detect "frozen efforts" (Laban, 1960) in still pictures. The opposite of "state" is the process of variations, upon which Lamb bases his notation, as we do.

STRAINING: A term for an "anal-sadistic" type of rhythm of tension-flow. Also used for the precursor of strength when it is accompanied by bound flow.

SUBORDINATION OF SHAPE-FLOW TO SHAPING IN SPACE: Flow- regulation in various parts of the body by which se- quence of shape-flow changes are controlled by shap- ing elements. For instance, lengthening and shorten- ing lose their independence when they are subordinated to rhythms of ascending and descending.

SUBORDINATION OF TENSION-FLOW TO EFFORT: Flow regulation by which sequences of tension-flow changes are adapted to the effort elements. For instance, rhythms of abruptness and graduality change their timing when these attributes are used as impetus for acceleration and deceleration.

SUBSYSTEM: Components of a movement system, represented
on separate diagrams in the profile. In system 1
(represented on the left side of the profile) there
are three subsystems: tension-flow-attributes, elements
of precursors of effort and elements of effort. Theo-
retically, tension-flow rhythms are a subsystem in
system 1, but practically we do not use it as one because it cannot yet be compared to any other subsystem.
In system 2 (represented on the right side of the profile) there are five subsystems: attributes of bipolar
and unipolar shape-flow, shape-flow design and elements
of shaping in directions and shaping in planes. Subsystem affinity and clashing, both in vertical and in
horizontal affinity, allow us to distinguish between
many compatibilities and imcompatibilities which neither
fall into the category of consonance-dissonance nor
matching-mismatching. See these headings.

SUDDEN: See precursors of effort.

SUPEREGO: A psychic structure which differentiates from
the ego during prelatency and becomes established in
latency (elementary school age). Its functions are
taken over from parental prohibitions and setting of
goals. However, it is also influenced by tendencies
taken over from the id. We distinguish between the
punitive versus permissive functions and the aspiring
versus discouraging functions of the superego. The
latter is subsumed under the heading "Ego-Ideal". The
id's influence on the superego is revealed in its
cruelty or negligence and in its grandiosity or
denigration.

SUSTAINED*: See effort.

SYMMETRICAL: See shape-flow.

SYSTEM: In the terminology used here, system refers to
a set of functions which have in common either
1) Dealings with internal and external reality,
through tension-flow, precursors of effort and effort, or 2) Dealings with objects through shape-flow
(bipolar and unipolar), shape-flow design, shaping
in directions and in planes.
    In psychoanalytic terminology, system refers to
a set of functions in a psychic structure, such as
the id, the ego or the superego. See intersystemic,
intrasystemic.

TEMPERAMENT: Refers to preferences for certain rhythms
and discharge-modes which are repeated more often
than others or have become incorporated into the body-
attitude. One can note such preferences for certain
attributes, their combinations and sequences in brief
spans of time; and tendencies of a similar kind can
be observed in larger spans of time. For instance,
abrupt beginning and stopping can be seen in brief
activities or they can preface and end longer periods.
A gradual increase in tension can be observed in a

Temperament cont.

brief movement phrase, but it can **also** be seen on a
long term basis, with heights of intensity reaching
their peaks during certain periods of the day or the
night.

TENSION-FLOW: Pertains to rhythms of tension-flow and
the attributes that regulate them. Rhythms of tension-
flow reflect our bodily needs and they are guided by
our wishes. We have no direct control over tension-
flow rhythms, but we can change them by regulating
tension-flow attributes. These are put into the
service of feelings concerned with matters of safety
versus danger. Tension-flow is a manifestation of
elasticity which is ubiquitous in animate matter. In
humans, it can be noted in the fetus, the newborn,
the child and the adult. Tension-flow attributes are
genetic forerunners of precursors of effort and effort,
and the latter incorporate tension-flow into their
sphere of operation.

The elements of tension-flow are free and bound,
the former acting as releaser and the latter as re-
strainer of movement. Neutral flow pertains to the
state of muscles (in movement and rest) in which
elasticity is decreased. See neutral flow.

In addition to the two basic elements of bound and
free flow, we note the following attributes (intensity
factors):

    a) Those affined with "fighting" effort elements
       and associated with states of frustration are:
       even level of tension; high intensity of tension;
       and abrupt change of tension.
    b) Those affined with "indulging" elements of ef-
       fort and associated with states of satiation
       or relief, are: adjustment of tension-level;
       low intensity of tension; and gradual change
       of tension.

The elements of tension, bound and free, are interrelated with feelings of caution and ease. Attributes
of tension-flow reflect a variety of feelings, simple
or complex. Preferred patterns of tension-flow are
the substrate of a person's temperament. Examples:
Even flow of tension predominates in people who appear
unruffled, phlegmatic or even-tempered. Flow-adjust-
ment predominates in those who are pliant, twisting,
restless or shy. High intensity of tension is the
mark of excitable people, easy to anger, easy to
frustrate or else living in a continuous state of high
excitation. Low intensity is noted in low-keyed, depressed or calm, not easily frustrated people. Abruptness of tension-increase and-decrease is a sign of
impulsivity, impatience, jumpiness, irritability or
alertness. Gradual increases and decreases of tension

are characteristic of deliberate people who need long preparations before they can become involved or before they can give up their involvement.

It should be noted that a temperament can express itself in the body attitude, with a persistence of a quality through movement and rest. In such an instance, there would be only few repetitions of this quality and the diagram in the profile would show a small area of variations in this particular attribute. More frequently, the quality which permeates the body-attitude is also subject to frequent variations, so that one can see a large area of the corresponding attribute in the diagram. Lastly, in some cases there is a relative absence of the particular temperamental quality in the body attitude, but its variations are many. An example of the latter is a person looking heavy or strong and surprisingly displaying many light movements. See tension-flow, temperament.

UNIPOLAR: See shape-flow.
VEHEMENT: See precursor of effort
VERTICAL: See shaping in planes.
VISION-DRIVE*: See effort, drives.
WIDENING: See shape-flow.
WRINGING*: See effort, basic.

REFERENCES

Abraham, K. (1924). A short study of the development of the libido, viewed in light of mental disorders. Selected Papers on Psycho-Analysis. London: Hogarth Press, pp. 418-501.

Alpert, A., Neubauer, P. B., & Weil, A. P. (1956). Unusual variations in drive endowment. The Psychoanalytic Study of the Child, 11:125-163. New York: International Universities Press.

Balint, M. (1959). Thrills and Regressions. New York: International Universities Press.

Berlowe, J. B. (1972). Movement Profile Scoring. New York: Child Development Research.

Dell, C. (1970). Primer for Movement Description. New York: Dance Notation Bureau.

Freud, A. (1965). Normality and Pathology in Childhood: Assessment of Development. New York: International Universities Press.

Freud, S. (1915). Instincts and their vicissitudes. Standard Edition, 14:109-140. London: Hogarth Press, 1957.

_____ (1917). Introductory Lectures on Psychoanalysis. Standard Edition, 15 & 16. London: Hogarth Press, 1963.

_____ (1920). Beyond the pleasure principle. Standard Edition, 18:3-64. London: Hogarth Press, 1955.

_____ (1924). The economic problem of masochism. Standard Edition, 19:157-172. London: Hogarth Press, 1961.

Fries, M. & Woolf, P. J. (1958). Some hypotheses on the role of the congenital activity type in personality and development. Psychoanalytic Study of the Child, 8:48-62. New York: International Universities Press.

References

Gottschalk, L. A. (1968). Some applications of the psychoanalytic concept of object-relatedness: Preliminary studies on a human relations content analysis scale applicable to verbal samples. Comprehensive Psychiatry, 9:608-619.

Greenacre, P. (1954). Problems of infantile neurosis. Psychoanalytic Study of the Child, 9:18-24.

Hartmann, H. (1939). Ego Psychology and the Problem of Adaptation. New York: International Universities Press, 1958.

Hermann, I. (1963). Die Theorie des primaren Anklammerungstriebes. Munich: Stefan Geroly.

Jacobson, E. (1964). Anxiety and Tension Control: A Physiologic Approach. Philadelphia: J. B. Lippincott.

Kestenberg, J. S. (1953). History of an autistic child. J. Child Psychiatry, 2:5-52.

_____ (1965). The role of movement patterns in development I: Rhythms of movement; II: Flow of tension and effort. Psychoanalytic Quarterly, 34:1-36, 34:517-63.

_____ (1967). The role of movement patterns in development III: The control of shape. Psychoanalytic Quarterly, 36:356-409.

_____ (1967b). The Role of Movement Patterns in Development, Vol. 1. New York: DNB Press, 1971.

_____ (1969). Problems of technique of child analysis in relation to the various developmental stages: Prelatency. Psychoanalytic Study of the Child, 24:358-83.

_____ (1971). A developmental approach to disturbances of sex-specific identity. International Journal of Psychoanalysis, 52:99-102.

_____ (1974). Self, environment and objects. Unpublished.

_____ (1975). Children and Parents: Psychoanalytic Studies in Development. New York: Jason Aronson.

_____ (1976). Regression and reintegration in pregnancy. Journal of the American Psychoanalytic Association (supplement), 24:213-250.

_____ (1979). Ego-Organization in Obsessive-Compulsive Development. In M. Kanzer and J. Glenn (ed.) "Down-State Psychoanalytic Division 25th Anniversary Volume". New York: Aronson.

Kestenberg, J. S. & Buelte, A. (1977a). Prevention in infant therapy: Its relevance to the treatment of adults. I, Toward an understanding of mutuality. International Journal of Psychoanalytic Psychotherapy. New York: Aronson.

_____ (1977b). Prevention in infant therapy: Its relevance to the treatment of adults. II, Holding each other and holding oneself up. International Journal of Psychoanalytic Psychotherapy. New York: Aronson.

Kestenberg, J. S. & Marcus, H. (1979). Notes on bisexuality. In M. C. Coleman (ed.), The Self in Process Series. New York: Behavioral Publications.

Kestenberg, J. S. & Robbins. E. (1975). Rhythmicity in adolescence. In Children and Parents: Psychoanalytic Studies in Development. New York: Jason Aronson.

Kohut, H. (1971). The Analysis of the Self. New York: International Universities Press.

Laban, R. (1960). The Mastery of Movement. Second Edition. Revised by L. Ullmann. London: Macdonald & Evans.

Laban, R. & Lawrence, F. (1947). Effort. London: Macdonald & Evans.

Lamb, W. (1961). Correspondence Course in Movement Assessment. Unpublished.

Lamb, W. (1965). Posture and Gesture. London: Gerald Duckworth.

Lamb, W. & Turner, D. (1969). Management Behavior. New York: International Universities Press.

Lomax, A., Bartenieff, I. and Paulay, F. (1967). Choreometrics. In A. Lomax (ed.), Folksong Style and Culture. New York: American Association for the Advancement of Science.

Mahler, M. (1968). On Human Symbiosis and the Vicissitudes of Individuation. New York: International Universities Press.

References

North, M. (1972). <u>Personality Assessment Through Movement</u>. London: Macdonald & Evans.

Ramsden, P. (1973). <u>Top Team Planning. A Study of the Power of Individual Motivation in Management</u>. New York: John Wiley.

Reich, W. (1927). <u>Die Funktion des Orgasmus</u>. Vienna: Int. Psa. Verlag.

Ruckmick, C. A. (1923). The rhythmical experience from the systematic point of view. <u>American Journal of Psychology</u>, 39.

Stern, M. (1951). Pavor nocturnus. <u>International Journal of Psychoanalysis</u>, 32:302-309.

Werner, H. (1948). <u>Comparative Psychology of Mental Development</u>. New York: International Universities Press.

Winnicott, D. W. (1957). <u>Mother and Child</u>. New York: Basic Books, Inc.